Trance Formed Body

Trance Formed Body

Control Your Weight, Size, and Shape with Self-Hypnosis

Copyright
© 2015, Robert P. DeGroot, M.Ed., D.C.H.
All rights reserved.

Disclaimer
This book is not a substitute for conventional medical or mental health advice and care.

DO NOT READ THIS BOOK to someone who is driving or operating equipment that requires their full attention.

DO NOT READ THIS BOOK when your attention is required elsewhere such as cooking, sitting in your car with the engine running, laying in the sun, caring for children or many other situations that lengthy distraction could prove hazardous.

Every reasonable effort has been made to ensure the accuracy of information and the processes incorporated into this text. However, even with this effort, understand that any application of the methods provided herein is at the reader's discretion.

Published by
Sales Training International, 5781 Cape Harbour Dr. Unit 607
Cape Coral, Florida 33915
www.TranceFormedBody.com

Trance Formed Body: Use self-hypnosis to change your weight, size, and shape.
ISBN: 978-0-9864058-0-8
1. Weight loss self-hypnosis. 2. Hypnosis scripts to control weight. 3. Self-help weight control.

R060217

Contents

About the Author iv
Preface v
Chapter 1 Face Your Frustrations 1
Chapter 2 Identify Your Control Mechanisms 5
Chapter 3 Experience Your Natural Trance State 19
Chapter 4 Create Your New Body Image 38
Chapter 5 Reinforce Your New Body Image 61
Chapter 6 Undermine Your Belly Fat 77
Chapter 7 Discover Your Motivators 97
Chapter 8 Supercharge Your Goals 113
Chapter 9 Create New Attitudes 128
Chapter 10 Uncover Your Blocker Beliefs 143
Chapter 11 Replace Your Blocker Beliefs 170
Chapter 12 Harness Your Fears 185
Chapter 13 Access Your Internal Resources 207
Chapter 14 Win the Mental Game 225
APPENDIX 235
    Blink Induction 236
    Deepening Staircase: Body Sculpting 239
    Work with the Full-Length Mirrors 243
    Power-up Motivator Beliefs into Attitudes 245
    Replace Obsolete Beliefs with Supportive Beliefs / Attitudes 245
    Redirect Fears and Create Supportive Beliefs / Attitudes 246
    Reawakening Staircase: Body Sculpting / Count up 247

About the Author

Dr. Robert P. DeGroot earned his Bachelor of Arts degree in Psychology and Master of Education in school psychology from Texas State University. He earned his Doctor of Clinical Hypnotherapy degree from the American Institute of Hypnotherapy.

Bob is certified by the American Board of Hypnotherapy and holds Fellow status in the American Psychotherapy Association.

He's a best-selling author, counselor, consultant, trainer and instructional designer. His first book about sales psychology led to the founding of Sales Training International.

In addition to *Trance Formed Body*, Bob has written over 70 instructor led training manuals, 50 Web-based training courses, and 42 eBooks.

For more information: www.BobDeGroot.com

Preface

Trance is the easiest way to open a direct communication channel with your subconscious mind which ultimately controls your weight, size, and shape. Now with the guidance provided in this book, you will learn how to use self-hypnosis inductions and deepening techniques to access your own naturally occurring trance state.

While in trance, you will work with the six primary areas that make it such a seemingly hopeless struggle to get and keep the body you want. Let's quickly review these areas.

First, your subconscious mind is maintaining the body weight, size, and shape you've got now because that's the current image it has of you. With trance, you can quickly embed a new picture of the body you want, so it knows what to build and maintain for you.

Second, under stress, your body generates an insulin spike that turns calories to fat and a cortisol spike that puts the fat on your belly. You can significantly diminish and even stop this effect with simple coping strategies both in and out of trance.

Third, the subconscious beliefs that sustain your motivators may not strong enough to compel you to make the right choices. These beliefs need to be strengthened into attitudes that will automatically guide your decisions.

Fourth, you hold certain once-useful, but now-obsolete, core beliefs operating at the subconscious level that blocks your ability to change your weight, size, and shape. They must be replaced by supportive beliefs and then powered-up into attitudes.

Fifth, you have a biologically based fear center that perceives weight change as threatening. Redirect the power of your fear center and retrain it or it will fight hard to reverse any success you have changing your weight, size, and shape.

Sixth, you have many internal resources such as courage and self-control that must be singled out, powered-up, and made a part of your lifestyle to make it much easier to get and maintain the body you want.

This unusual book is written like a novel using dialogue format. It tells the story of two couples working with a hypnotherapist to learn how to use self-hypnosis to get the bodies they want. Simply read along and go into trance with them to learn how to use self-hypnosis to access your natural trance state to get the body you want.

The characters and conversations are fictional. They are designed to answer common questions about hypnosis, address issues with weight control, and to keep you engaged while you learn how to use self-hypnosis to achieve your own weight, size, and shape goals.

The information about weight control psychology, hypnosis, trance inductions, deepening techniques, and trance work are real and wonderfully effective when completed according to the instructions given. Further, to enhance your feelings of comfort with hypnosis, you'll do it all with your eyes open using time-tested self-hypnosis techniques.

You can add, modify, or delete the suggestions in this book to better meet your specific needs. In fact, in some of the hypnosis scripts you'll read, there are fill in the blanks templates designed for you to personalize the suggestions to increase their effectiveness with you.

Thank you for purchasing this book to facilitate your journey into your subconscious mind to help you get and keep the body you want.

Bob DeGroot

Chapter 1 Face Your Frustrations

Jean stared into her closet and shrieked, "I can't take it anymore. I'm so fat. None of my clothes fit."

John startled but quickly understood as he slouched in his oversized chair with his belt unbuckled and his pants loosened. He, too, was extremely uncomfortable with his size and said with an intensity that surprised him, "I hear you. Just look at me. I'm the same way."

She walked over and sat across from him. With tears in her eyes and pleading in her voice, she asked, "What are we going to do?"

John looked at her with concern but could only sigh.

"We can't keep going on like this," she said. "We've got to do something. I don't want to end up with any of those terrible conditions overweight people get. On top of that, I am really beginning to resent how people look at us."

"We've tried just about every diet out there," he said. "I'm not sure what we should do."

"I know," she said. "We initially get excited and then after a while, we just stop doing it."

"And our weight goes back up," he said.

"I just don't think I can go through that again," she said.

"Me neither," he said. "I tell you what let's do. We're smart people. Maybe we can figure out our own plan. We know what we need to do and we're already eating healthy foods."

"Yeah, I know," she said. "But for some reason, we just can't take any pounds off."

"So what are we missing?" he asked.

"I don't know, I don't know," she said. "But it's got to be something mental or emotional or motivational or something else entirely. I just know there has got to be something we've completely overlooked."

"Jean, darling, we'll figure it out. But right now it's pretty late, and so before we get really down on ourselves, we need to call it a night and start fresh tomorrow."

John and Jean drug themselves out of their seats, got ready, and fell into bed, both thinking about what it could possibly be that they missed during all their attempts to get control of their weight.

The next day Jean came home from work and said, "John, you'll never guess who I had lunch with today."

Holding his fingers to his forehead he said, "Yes, I can. It was Betty."

"How did you know?" she asked.

"I'm psychic," he laughed. "Not really, she just called and told me about your lunch and said she's got great news but she wouldn't tell me. She said that would spoil the surprise."

Jean was already dialing before John finished his sentence.

"Hi, Betty, it's Jean, I hear you have some good news?" she asked.

"Oh, I'm so excited," Betty said. "There is this fun couple who live on the first floor of our building. We've known them for a long time. We see them all the time at the condo social events and out walking or getting the mail, but I never really knew what he did."

"But now you do?"

"Turns out, when I was getting our mail, I talked with a neighbor about trying to lose a few pounds, and she said I should talk to the hypnotist on the first floor."

"I never thought about using hypnosis, but I guess we need to find out if it can help," Jean said. "Who is he?"

"Dr. Bob DeGroot. He knows about psychology and hypnosis."

"That's great," Jean said. "Maybe he can just hypnotize us to lose weight."

"I don't know about that," Betty said. "But I was just so excited, I called him and he said he'd be happy to meet with us and answer any questions we have."

"Thank you so much, Betty. I owe you big time on this one," Jean said.

"That's all well and good, but here's the deal. Ed and I want to be there," Betty said.

"Really?" Jean asked.

"You know we've been trying everything we can to lose weight," Betty said. "We've even thought about surgery. But we're open to exploring other options before we take such a drastic step."

"I didn't know," Jean said. "Of course, you can be there. You know Bob, and if he can help, it would make sense for the four of us to work together. Maybe we can even keep each other from those desserts we eat at work."

"You're on," Betty said.

"What do you know about this guy professionally?" Jean asked.

"Ed did a quick search and it turns out he's a Doctor of Clinical Hypnotherapy with all sorts of other credentials in psychology and counseling," Betty said.

"How soon do you think we could meet with him?" Jean asked.

"Would tomorrow evening around 6 o'clock at our condo be early enough?" Betty asked.

"First," she said, "let me check with John to let him know what we're planning. Could you hold on for a minute?"

"Of course," Betty said.

Jean called out, "Hey, John."

"What?" he asked.

"There's a Doctor of Clinical Hypnotherapy –
"A what?" John interrupted.

"A hypnotist," Jean said. "Betty and Ed know him because he lives in their condo building. Betty talked with him, and he said he'd be happy to meet with us about our weight problem. Betty said she could set it up for tomorrow evening around 6 o'clock at their place. What about it? Are you up for it?" she asked.

"With you and Betty ganging up, do I have a choice?" he asked.

"Ha, what do you think?" Jean said to John as she turned back to the phone.

"OK," Jean said. "Tomorrow evening will be good for us."

"I'll call Dr. Bob back to firm up the time," Betty said.

"What can we bring?" Jean asked.

"Nothing at all," Betty said. "You know how much I love hosting our little get-togethers."

"Then," Jean said, "I'll fill John in on Dr. Bob's background, and we'll see you tomorrow."

Chapter 2 Identify Your Control Mechanisms

The next day, John and Jean arrived early at Betty and Ed's condo. They spent a few minutes settling in before there was a knock on the door.

Ed jumped up and welcomed Dr. Bob DeGroot.

Introductions went quickly, and everyone got comfortable.

Betty spoke first. "Doctor, can you just hypnotize us to lose weight?" she asked.

"Betty, everyone," he said. "I'm retired. Call me Bob."

Heads nodded.

"Now to answer your question," Bob said. "I can teach you how to use self-hypnosis with your eyes open so you can read yourself into a trance, read your own weight, size, and shape-related suggestions, and then bring yourself back out of the trance."

"That would be great," Betty said.

"As I understand from Ed and Betty, you've all tried different diets that seemed to work well initially, but over time and for various reasons, you weren't able to stay with them," Bob said.

"Yes," Jean said. "It's like I was telling John. We know what to do, but no matter what, we just can't seem to do it over the long haul."

John, Betty, and Ed each nodded their heads in agreement.

"That's fairly common," Bob said. "There are six primary areas controlled by your subconscious mind that can cause that to happen and interfere with your long-term success."

"We're all ears," Ed said.

"Does everybody have a weight goal in mind?" Bob asked.

Heads nodded and Ed volunteered, "I'd like to weigh 175 pounds."

"I want you to think about your number and tell me what that physically looks like for you," Bob said. "Now don't respond out loud. Just answer the question to yourselves."

Silence.

"What do you mean?" Betty asked. "I couldn't tell by my number what I would look like. I hadn't thought about it that way.

"Well," Bob said. "In the long run, your subconscious mind controls your weight, size, and shape. The last image it holds of you is what gives you the bodies you have now."

"If that's the case," Ed said, "doesn't my goal of 175 pounds cover that?"

"Not really," Bob said. "The subconscious mind does better with pictures, imagery, symbols, and emotions than it does with numbers. That's one of the main reasons why you want to clarify exactly what you want your body to look like. If it helps, you can use pictures of yourself at that size and shape."

"My goal of weighing 125 pounds means what then?" Jean asked.

"Unless you can clearly see what that physically looks and feels like," Bob said, "it's really too fuzzy for your subconscious mind to work with. It's easier for your subconscious mind to recognize size and shape than it is to perceive 125 pounds. If you can't imagine what that looks and feels like, how can your subconscious mind create that for you?"

"Yeah," Jean said. "I understand."

"The more the subconscious experiences and accepts the design, structure, size, texture, color, temperature, taste, smell, sound, and any emotion you might associate with your body image, then the more real it becomes," Bob said. "The more real that image becomes, the more it's possible for you to

Identify Your Control Mechanisms

achieve it. So your first goal will be to get the subconscious mind to accept and believe as real, this new image of the size and shape you want that's right for your body's height and frame."

"Frame?" Betty asked.

"Skeletal bone structure," Bob said. "Some people have big bones and some people have smaller ones. That would, of course, affect weight and shape goals."

"Uh huh," Betty said.

"Use one of those online calculators or charts that take your height and frame into consideration to find out what your weight range should be," Bob said. "You can use this for reference to help you zero in on images."

"We can do that," Ed said.

"After you've done that," Bob said, "we probably won't talk much about weight in terms of pounds but rather focus on what the subconscious mind can use to help you."

"And that's size and shape," Jean said. "I think we've got that now."

"Stress is another area that can stop your efforts cold," Bob said. "When you're stressed, your body pumps a lot of chemicals such as insulin to convert calories into fat and cortisol to put the fat on your bellies."

"Oh, that's where I think I'll need the most help," Betty said.

"I think she speaks for all of us," Ed said.

"It's unfortunate that as soon as you start making progress, stress can step in and add fat where you least want it to go," Bob said.

"We should start with that," John said.

"I'll put it early in the process," Bob said. "After that, the next area that you'll need to deal with at the subconscious level has to do with your motivation for achieving your weight, size, and shape goals."

"I think we're all pretty motivated or we wouldn't be sitting here," John said.

"That's true," Bob said. "Now let me ask you, with previous weight loss programs, when you hit the tough times, were those motivators strong enough to see you through?"

"Now that you put it that way, I guess not," Betty said.

"A lot of times the process breaks down when the motivation fades," Bob said.

"No doubt that could be part of the problem we're having," John said.

"What you'll need to do then, "Bob said, "is look to your subconscious mind to discover both the obvious and the hidden motivators and get them directly connected to your size and shape goals. Once you find them, you'll test their strength and then if you need to, I'll show you how to power them up to maximum strength so they have enough force to carry you through."

"That would be awesome," Jean said.

"That sounds like something we need," John said.

"I'm in," Ed said. "Let's go."

"Ed," John said. "I think we all want to hear about the other areas."

Smiling, Bob said, "Yes, there are just a few more issues operating at the subconscious level that can put a stop to your efforts that you don't want to overlook."

"We're all ears," Ed said.

"Everyone holds certain core beliefs that operate at the subconscious level. These core beliefs guide your thinking and behavior in all areas of your life, including eating."

"There are subconscious beliefs that say 'eat?'" Betty asked.

Identify Your Control Mechanisms

"Yes," Bob said. "As you've discovered, most diets, when followed carefully, do tend to work for a while but then as soon as you are no longer 'consciously' vigilant, your subconscious mind steps back in, takes over and returns you to what it 'believes' your weight should be. These mostly obsolete beliefs that are wrong for you now, still control your weight, size, and shape and will continue to do so until you change them. I call them blocker beliefs."

"Can you give me a specific example?" Jean asked.

"Let's do two quick examples," Bob said. "The first is how your subconscious mind takes control when you are not focusing on the task directed by the conscious mind. That could be anything such as changing your pattern of breathing to changing your pattern of eating. And the second example will be with a specific blocker belief."

"This should be interesting," Ed said.

"Let's go then," Bob said. "Take a deep breath through your nose, hold it, and now let it out slowly through your mouth. Again, take a deep breath through your nose, hold it, and now let it out slowly through your mouth. Now continue to breathe that way while we talk about one of the blocker beliefs.

"Suppose you believe that you must clean your plate of all the food," Bob said. "That may have been important when you were young, but now it's wrong for you. This means you'll need to modify that obsolete belief to something along the lines of, 'I only eat what I need and throw the rest away.'"

"Oh, that would be so hard to do," Betty said.

"Wasting food is tough," Bob said. "That's why I used that example. But doesn't that point to another one of your core beliefs?"

"Yes," Betty said. "That's been ingrained in me since I was very young. Maybe some of these childhood beliefs like believing in an actual tooth fairy need to change."

"So you'll need to work on different strategies and supportive beliefs to help change that counterproductive belief that blocks you from achieving your goal to something completely acceptable. If you don't, your subconscious mind will make sure you eat everything on your plate."

"But if these supportive beliefs are like positive affirmations, we've used them repeatedly in the past. They didn't take hold," Betty said.

Bob smiled and said, "That's because you've been trying to change them at the conscious level rather than at the subconscious level where they operate. Hypnosis will help you communicate those ideas or new beliefs directly with the subconscious mind."

"So they have to be changed where they work?" John asked.

"Yes," Bob said. "And by the way, how are you breathing? Are you breathing in through your nose, holding it, and then breathing out through your mouth?"

"I think not," Ed said.

"What happened?" Bob asked.

"We got distracted by …" Ed said.

"Yes, Ed," Bob said. "Once you get distracted from your diet, your subconscious mind takes over and returns your behavior to what it knows and believes you should do, which includes eating more."

"Your point is well taken," John said.

"And the next thing that can sabotage us?" Ed asked.

"Oh, you'll like this one," Bob said. "There is a wonderful pair of biological brain structures called the amygdalae. From prehistoric times they've used fear to keep you safe. Although they do other things, for weight, size, and shape control, what you need to be concerned with is their fear function."

"I don't see how we're afraid to lose weight," John said.

Identify Your Control Mechanisms

"Let's explore that notion," Bob said. "When these brain parts, we'll just call the fear center, sense a situation that could be a threat to your survival, they react to keep you out of harm's way. There is no thinking, just reacting. They help you jump out of the way of a car coming at you or catch yourself when you trip. It's all reactive, and that's a good thing."

"I can see that," Ed said. "But I'm not sure how that applies to what we're trying to do."

"When your weight control actions cause changes that are perceived as threats, you'll have a fight on your hands every moment of the day," Bob said.

"How can what we're doing to lose weight be perceived as a threat?" Betty asked.

"For one, a drop in the number of calories you're consuming could be perceived by parts of your primitive brain that you're entering a time of extreme scarcity of food and that could lead to starvation and ultimately death," Bob said. "Or, even changing the types of foods you're eating or changing your activities. Any of these changes could elicit subconscious hyper-vigilance to a possible threat that would cause this fear function to slow down or even stop your efforts."

"We're not talking about starving ourselves, are we?" Ed asked.

"Maybe, maybe not," Bob said. "But you have something called the starvation reflex. This is a response to severely restricting the numbers of calories you take in versus what your body needs.

"If you do this longer than a couple of days, your body thinks it's experiencing a famine and begins to slow your metabolism and hoard calories to survive. So when this happens, you don't use fat for energy. Your body wants to store it to use later, to keep you from starving to death, and that's how you could gain weight."

"I know about that," John said. "The last diet we tried made me feel like I was starving. I was hungry all the time."

"So what happened when you decided not to starve yourself?" Bob asked.

"We did this for almost a month, and when we gave up on that plan, it seemed like we couldn't get enough to eat," John said.

"And that's the other side of the starvation reflex," Bob said. "As soon as you increase the number of calories you take in, your body decides this famine is over and decides to add some extra fat to prepare for the next famine. It seems like the longer you're on one of these type diets, the longer it takes for your body to recalibrate what it needs to satisfy your hunger."

"Well, that explains why we gain more weight than we lose after we ease up on strictly following the diet or when we change to a new one," John said. "I'll bet that's what causes yo-yo dieting results."

"That could be part of it," Bob said.

"Oh my," Betty said. "This fear center sounds like it can be hard to deal with."

"It can be," Bob said. "But the good news is that you can harness the power of your fear center and use it to your advantage. You can also retrain it so that it won't fight you but rather support the change you need to achieve your goals."

"That's good to know," Betty said.

"To be on the safe side so you don't trigger the fear center," Bob said, "target your fat reduction goals at one to two pounds a week. One pound is 3,500 calories."

"I thought I could lose fat faster than that," Ed said.

"You can," Bob said. "But in addition to risking the starvation reflex, you might set an unrealistic expectation which is the first stage of burnout."

Identify Your Control Mechanisms

"I think Jean and I experienced that more than a few times," John said. "We'd start with big expectations to lose a lot of weight fast and then we'd hit a plateau, get frustrated, and give up."

"Thank you," Bob said. "You just named all four stages of burnout."

"Are we going to have to count calories?" Jean asked. "It's such a hassle."

"It would be a good idea to know how many calories you need to maintain the body you've got versus how many calories you need to maintain the body you want," Bob said. "That way you can begin to gradually reduce the number of calories you consume. There are calculators and charts online you can use to get an idea of what that would be, as well as, the levels you should target."

"Anyway you look at it," Ed said, "we're going to have to consume fewer calories than we use."

"Yeah," John said. "I guess we're going to have to do that."

"Again," Bob said, "you really just want to get a picture of the amount of food it takes to maintain the body you've got and the amount it would take to maintain the body you want. You might keep a daily list of what, when, and how much you eat to see if there are any patterns that could be interfering with achieving your goal. If there are, most of the time they're pretty obvious."

"I can see how that would tell us if we're really starting to adjust or if we're really just kidding ourselves," John said.

"Our minds are pretty good at getting us to believe we're not eating any more than we have in the past," Bob said. "But most of the time that's just not true. It all adds up and adds up fast.

"For example, you might think you've hit a plateau, or maybe start to think that what you're doing isn't working, or some other challenge is stopping your progress, when in fact you've just started to increase how much you're eating," Bob said. "Or you might be changing the types of foods you're eating for higher calorie versions, or you could be decreasing the amount of physical activity you're getting."

"Or all of the above," Ed said. "And I guess we won't know for sure unless we begin to track what we're doing now."

"What you want is to get a good idea about your eating patterns and portion sizes," Bob said. "Keep a close watch on it, at least until you've reached your goal. You really want to know the difference of how much you're consuming now and how much you would consume at your target weight. Awareness of this difference is critical."

"I never thought about how much I would be eating when I reach my goal," John said. "But I guess if we don't recalibrate to what that amount looks like, we might never get there."

"John," Jean said, "you're the lab guy, why don't you divide the food tonight based on how much we eat now and put that on one plate and then on another plate put the amount we will be eating when we get to our target weight."

"That's a great idea," Ed said. "We'll do the same."

"If we have a week where we don't lose our pound," Betty said, "I guess that would be a good time to start tracking it for the next week so we can see what needs to be adjusted."

"That's it exactly," Bob said. "The objective is to keep gradually rolling back the amount of food you consume each week until you start reducing your weight. If you want, you can do this without changing your current level of physical activity so you know it's the calorie reduction that's working."

"How often should we do this?" Ed asked.

Identify Your Control Mechanisms

"I would suggest you adjust weekly so you can stabilize at that level before reducing the calorie levels again," Bob said. "If you stall or aren't getting the results you want, you would first check to see that you really are eating what you thought you were and if so, you could increase your physical activity levels or roll back more calories."

"I can live with four pounds a month coming off permanently," Jean said. "That way I won't feel guilty buying new clothes because I know they'll be used for a long time. I really want to wear skinny jeans."

"That's a good example of focusing on size and shape," Bob said. "The goal is to restore your body to what it would naturally and normally look like without this extra fat so that you can wear the types and sizes of clothes that are right for your body's frame."

"Bob," Ed said. "I'm picking up that you steer away from using terms like losing weight. Am I right?"

"Yes," Bob said. "I prefer to move in a positive direction and focus on what you want rather than what you don't want."

"How so?" Ed asked.

"In many situations, the subconscious mind doesn't recognize or comprehend negative words so it's better to avoid them altogether," Bob said.

"What do you mean by negative words?" Betty asked.

"Instructions that say 'don't' or 'won't,'" Bob said. "For example, young children spend much of their time in trance, so what happens when you say to a child, 'don't fall down?'"

"Oh," Betty said, "they almost always fall down. I guess it's the same when you say, 'don't touch that - it's hot.'"

"Yes," Bob said. "That's because, in trance, the subconscious mind didn't process the word 'don't' and only heard the command to 'fall down,' or 'touch that.' By the way, did you notice that you can create a clear mental picture or image of 'fall down,' or 'touch that?'"

"Weird for the kids, but I can see it happening," John said.

"So we want to use words that create a picture for the subconscious mind?" Jean asked.

"The more detailed the better," Bob said.

"But doesn't weight loss speak to that?" Ed asked.

"It does," Bob said. "But while doing that, it also brings up images we don't want that could interfere with your size and shape goals."

"Explain please," Ed said.

"Suppose you heard that a friend had lost 40 pounds. A question that might come to mind would be, 'was that intentional or did illness play a role?'"

"Oh, I would definitely think that," Betty said.

"We don't want to send mixed messages to the subconscious about what your true goal is and that is to reduce the excess fat stored in your bodies," Bob said. "You don't want to lose muscle and bone in the process, so giving the subconscious mind the clearest instructions you can is critical."

"Apparently to the subconscious," Ed said, "losing weight is losing weight, muscle, and bone or whatever."

"As a side issue," Bob said, "what do you normally do when you lose something?"

"Try to find it and get it back," John said.

"Does anybody here like losing things?" Bob asked.

"I think I see where you're going with this," Ed said. "Losing weight is still losing, and we don't like to lose so there might be more mixed messages running around in the background."

"So for the sake of minimizing mixed messages," Bob said, "we'll keep the conversations focused on getting what you want."

Identify Your Control Mechanisms

"Jean and I talked about wanting to tone our muscles so they keep us from the saggy baggy look," John said.

"Getting that toned body look simply means removing the fat that's covering the muscles you've got so they show through and define your look," Bob said.

"How do we talk about what we want to do then?" Jean asked.

"Focus on your size and shape goals," Bob said. "You want to imagine your body as slim, trim, and physically fit. Those are images the subconscious mind can work with so you want to keep those in front of you."

"Now I understand," Jean said.

"When your subconscious mind believes that this imagined slim, trim, and physically fit body is your true body size and shape," Bob said, "it will automatically begin to guide you to act, eat, and move to create this body at the physical level."

"You know," Jean said, "there are times when I just don't seem to be strong enough to stick with something I know is working. Is there something you can add into what we're going to do to help with that?"

"Yes," Bob said. "That's the final area we'll explore. Everyone has internal resources such as passion, courage, and desire that will come out when you care about something deeply enough."

"Can we start there?" Betty asked.

"Since you've all been down the road of disappointment before," Bob said, "I'm going to suggest we use this component at the end to cover anything else that might interfere with your long-term success.

"I'm beginning to understand how the subconscious mind is maintaining our body's size and shape," Ed said. "What I'd like to know is how hypnosis will help us make the changes we need to make with our subconscious minds."

Chapter 3 Experience Your Natural Trance State

"Good transition," Bob said. "I think this is a good time to start to understand the basics of hypnosis. That way you'll be able to make an informed decision about using it to help you achieve your weight, size, and shape goals."

"You might have noticed I'm a little skeptical," Ed said. "So I really need to be more comfortable with this."

"I'm glad to hear that," Bob said. "That'll help make sure we don't miss anything."

"Ed," Betty said. "Behave."

"I'm with Ed on this," John said. "I've seen a hypnosis show and have some questions about how they got those people to do those crazy things."

"To begin with," Bob said, "stage hypnosis has but one purpose and that is to entertain. To understand what's happening on the stage, we'll need to take some time to understand hypnosis for what it really is."

"OK," John said. "But I still want to ask the questions."

"Absolutely," Bob said, "We'll get through all of those for sure."

"That'll help," John said.

"First and foremost is to understand that the trance state is as natural and normal as your wide awake or your sleeping states," Bob said. "For example, have you ever got caught up in a movie or a good book and felt emotions, excitement, and suspense?"

"All the time," Jean said. "I can really get carried away with some of the novels I'm reading and, boy, some movies open the floodgates of emotion."

"Me, too," Betty said.

"Uh huh," commented Ed and John almost in unison.

"Hey there now," Jean said. "You get as caught up in your action movies as much as I do in my chick flicks."

"See how easy it is to go into trance?" Bob asked.

"I guess so," John said.

"Let's look at couple more common trance events," Bob said. "Have you ever been so mentally focused on something that you missed your exit while driving? Or, how about arriving home and not remembering the trip?"

"Guilty as charged," Ed said.

"I played sports in college," John said. "Mostly downhill skiing and we were trained to practice by imagining going down the course executing each turn perfectly. It was easy to get caught up in that and lose all track of time. We called it getting into the zone."

"So there you have it," Bob said. "Each of you has experienced trance in different situations from reading a book to watching a movie to missing an exit, to competitive skiing. Whether you call it getting in the zone, hypnosis, or trance, they're all the same thing."

"Are you saying we went into trance when we did that?" Jean asked.

"Sure," Bob said. "Again, trance is a naturally occurring state in which you are able to bypass the internal reality check function of your conscious mind. This reality check would tell you that the characters in the novel you're reading or the movie you're watching aren't real. But what fun is that?"

Ed took in a deep breath and let it out as he said nothing but, "Oh, boy."

"There are really just two conditions that are required for hypnosis to occur," Bob said. "First, we have to get by this reality checker I just mentioned so it doesn't interfere by telling us what's real and what's imagined. And second, we need to selectively choose supporting evidence that what we're imaging is real, at least to the subconscious mind."

"What do you mean by supporting evidence?" Ed asked.

"Suppose you were to imagine your body being at your targeted size and shape," Bob said. "As soon as you can imagine that, you've bypassed your reality checker."

"You got that right," Ed said.

"Funny," John said.

"That was quick," Bob said. After the laughter let up, Bob continued. "Imagining your body at the size and shape you want starts the process. When you then add something like seeing yourself wearing smaller size clothes for that image, you're selecting evidence to support your image of your body's new size and shape while at the same time ignoring equally valid contradictory evidence.

"In your mind, you're rationalizing that your smaller size clothes wouldn't fit unless what you imagined about your body size and shape is true. And because they do fit, it means your body must be that size and shape. That's the evidence the subconscious mind uses to know that it's real."

"It's like adding props to a stage show to make it more real for the audience," Betty said.

"That's it exactly," Bob said. "All those are aids to your imagination. Notice that there is evidence to the contrary as well. For example, the stage floor, the lighting, and other evidence of a conscious reality. What you do in hypnosis is enhance your ability to select the evidence that supports your imagined goal and ignore the rest."

"If that's supportive evidence I got it now," Ed said.

"The psychological process involved is called selective thinking," Bob said. "You select what you want to think about and what you want to let fade into the background.

"After you start seeing actual changes in your body's size and shape," Bob said, "the supporting evidence moves from your imagination to the realm of conscious reality."

"I think I better understand why we need to add the detail of what we're imagining," Jean said. "But first, don't we have to get past the reality checker you mentioned? How can we do that?"

"There are several ways to bypass it," Bob said. "I'll teach you what hypnotists call trance inductions to help you quickly go into trance."

"Good," Jean said. "But if we all go in and out of trance all the time, how do we do that without using a trance induction as you call it?"

"You could relax your mind so that it is no longer on alert for the unreal. Boredom does this when it leads to a trance called day dreaming," Bob said.

Jean started laughing and said, "I've been to many lectures that took me right into trance."

"Another way," Bob said, "is experiencing sudden strong emotions ranging from joy to fear that can jolt or stun the conscious mind out of action. You might instantly become speechless or motionless. Even momentary mental confusion can cause trance. It's the fight, flight, or freeze reaction."

"Kind of like the deer-in-the-headlight look,'" Ed said.

"That's it," Bob said. "Also physical pain automatically puts the person experiencing it into a trance. And there are some really powerful ways to use hypnosis to lessen the pain a person feels."

"Is that why some dentists use hypnosis?" Betty asked.

"Yes," Bob said. "Some people are too anxious or afraid of needles or are allergic to the medication used to numb the nerves. Hypnosis does a very efficient job in this setting, calming the person, removing fears, and controlling pain."

Experience Your Natural Trance State

"What about other ways we go into trance?" Ed asked.

"Rituals quickly bypass the reality checker, especially if led by an authority figure," Bob said. "Monotonous repetitions such as a drum beat, chanting, music, or even stripes on the highway can quickly numb the mind into a trance."

"Ed and I have a favorite song," Betty said. "We just get caught up in it and lost in our memories."

"Yes," Bob said. "Music we personally like can carry us mentally away to an imaginary place. And like you and Ed, a lot of people have a song that holds special meaning."

"We have a special song, too," Jean said. "And when we hear it we say, 'That's our song' and off we go into good memories and feelings. It's so real."

"Many people will play classical music softly in the background when they go into trance to help with full brain absorption and learning," Bob said.

"How's that?" Ed asked.

"It's a right brain or left brain thing," Bob said. "Left brain is logical and right brain is creative. The left brain reads, and the right brain imagines what's being read. The two sides of the brain are connected by a bundle of neurons. Music helps carry the logical to the imaginative."

"We don't have any classical music," Ed said. "How about something else?"

"Some easy listening music might do," Bob said. "But classical music is mathematically defined and has a positive effect on the mind and body. For now, better to stick with what the research, and in this case, personal experience shows works best."

"OK," John said. "Can we go back to getting past the reality checker?"

"Of course," Bob said. "One of my favorite ways to bypass the conscious mind's reality checker is to simply give yourself permission to do so by saying something like, 'Just imagine,' or, 'Pretend.'

"For kids, an easy induction is to say 'let's go to the land of make-believe and pretend.' That gives them permission to bypass reality. After that, you select the supporting evidence to create a story with lots of sensory stimulating picture words."

"Just that easy?" Ed asked.

"Usually yes," Bob said. "You can make it easier to set up the leap into a trance by giving yourself permission to imagine something strange and wonderful. For example, Alice went down a rabbit hole. That made it OK to believe all those strange things could be happening to Alice."

"So maybe it's not as complex as I'm making it out to be?" John asked.

"Actually, it's easier done than said," Bob said. "Let me demonstrate. Do you remember what a chalkboard is?"

Everyone nodded.

"Does anybody have any good memories about the chalkboard?" he asked. "Remember chalk dust getting on everything or remember writing on it?"

Heads nodded.

"Now just imagine yourself in a room with a chalkboard when someone scrapes their fingernails across it making that loud screeching sound that grates on your nerves. See it, hear it, feel it. Notice how this causes a shiver down your spine."

Everyone groaned. John's eyes went wide and then he shook his shoulders.

"Just to be sure, let's do another example," Bob said. "Here we are in Betty and Ed's home. You know the refrigerator is in the next room. But now for just a moment let's pretend that you're standing in front of that refrigerator staring at the door. Take a deep breath and let it out to help you get that picture clearly in your mind. Everyone have it? You can nod when you've got it. Good.

"Now imagine opening the door and seeing a jar of cold juicy dill pickles. Watch as your hand takes that cold jar out of the refrigerator and sets it on the counter. Open the jar and reach in and take out a big juicy dill pickle. Feel the wet cold juices dripping onto your hand. Now bring it to your mouth and bite into this big, cold, juicy dill pickle. Feel the crunch as you bite into it. Taste it. Feel the cold dill juices running under your tongue. Smell it. Feel it chill your teeth."

"Enough," John said. "My salivary glands are hurting."

Everyone laughed and nodded in agreement. They had all experienced it.

Bob said, "Notice how that multi-sensory imagery of the pickle provided enough supportive evidence that it caused you to salivate, or how the fingernails on the chalkboard caused a shiver down your spine. Are either the chalkboard or the pickle right here right now?" he asked.

Heads shook no.

"Be clear that while neither the chalkboard nor the pickles are present, the physical effects occurred anyway," Bob said. "The subconscious mind doesn't do a very good job of distinguishing what's real and what's imagined. It has difficulty telling the difference between a real pickle and an imagined one."

"That's really amazing when you think about it," John said.

"What's so important to realize," Bob said, "is that just by imagining something with a lot supporting evidence using multi-sensory input that's not even present in your conscious reality, you can still get the subconscious mind to make physical changes in your body. Isn't that what you just demonstrated you could do?"

"We did, didn't we?" Betty said.

"In our earlier examples, we talked about having a physical and emotional reaction to the books and movies. The characters in the book and movie were not real, but rather creations of the author who was able to engage you so completely in the story that you imagined them to be real enough to feel emotions, shed tears, laugh, or have any number physical and emotional reactions," he said.

"That's hypnosis?" Betty asked.

"Sure is," Bob said. "Any time you imagine something that is not present in your conscious reality, and your body responds physically and emotionally as though your imagined world were real, you're in trance."

"Imagining some story put us in trance and caused our bodies to respond?" Jean asked.

"As soon as you narrowed your focus to selective elements and evidence of the story, you automatically began to discard other non-supportive evidence such as the exit signs in the theater," Bob said. "Out of everything bombarding your senses, you tend to select the evidence you want to believe at the moment and create your reality out of that."

"And just by being in trance and using our imaginations we can change our bodies?" John asked.

"Absolutely," Bob said. "You demonstrated that a couple of times already, haven't you?"

"I guess so," John said.

"Now think about the physical changes your subconscious mind could make to your body when you make it believe that it should be creating and maintaining a body that is slim and trim."

"Like salivating or shivering because that's the response you targeted with the imagery you presented," John said.

Bob nodded his head and said, "Once the subconscious mind believes something to be true, it will do what is necessary to cause that belief to come to be true in the world of conscious physical reality. Whether that's salivating from an imagined pickle or becoming slim and trim by imagining a different size and shape for your body."

"This is a little scary to me when you think about living some fantasy as though it's real," Betty said.

"Yeah," Ed said. "How do we know what's real then?" he asked.

"During your everyday waking state, the reality checker in your conscious mind functions to help you separate the imaginary from the real," Bob said.

"The conscious mind will keep the imaginary in the unreal bin," Ed said.

"That's right," Bob said. "Hypnosis helps you get around that. If you don't, it will get in your way with its reality detector on high alert and fight you before you even get started."

"What if I can't be hypnotized?" Ed asked.

"That's a good question," Bob said. "Not everyone can go into hypnosis all the time whenever they want. But everyone does go into trance from time-to-time whether they intend to or not. It's a normal state of being, just like dreaming when you're asleep."

"OK then, how would I know when I'm in trance?" Ed asked. "We weren't relaxed when we imagined the chalkboard or the pickle. I thought we had to go into deep relaxation in order to be in hypnosis. We didn't do that."

"Yeah," John said. "Everyone I've seen in a hypnosis stage show that was supposed to be in trance looked like they were sleeping or totally out of it."

"Relaxation is commonly used as a part of many hypnosis inductions because it makes a person less anxious and therefore more receptive to suggestion. But that's not necessary for hypnosis to occur. Think about our earlier examples of going into trance reading a book or watching an exciting movie. Were you relaxed, alert, or even tense?"

"I certainly wasn't going to sleep, that's for sure," Ed said.

"Relaxing the body and then relaxing the mind can be used as part of a hypnotic induction that will prepare you to bypass the reality checker. But again, relaxation is just one method to do this. When you're using self-hypnosis with relaxation and you're really tired, you could definitely drift off into a natural sleep."

"I like that idea," Jean said.

"If you were to observe a sleeping person and a person who used relaxation to go into trance," Bob said, "while they may look the same, there would be some very big differences. Studies using functional magnetic resonance imaging, better known as an fMRI, demonstrated that different parts of the brain were active when the person was in hypnosis than when they were in normal sleep.

"Another big difference is that you can do some pretty extraordinary things during hypnosis, such as complete anesthesia for the whole body or just parts of it, to changing core beliefs held deep in the subconscious mind. These things can't be done in ordinary sleep or ordinary waking state."

"What about controlling our minds during hypnosis?" Ed asked. "I see the people at the hypnosis show do some pretty amazing things, and it looks like the hypnotist is telling them what to do and they are helpless to do otherwise."

"The people who volunteer for those shows, of course, are highly motivated to do what the hypnotist tells them to do," he said. "But it's the power of their own minds that enables them to do those things, not the power of the hypnotist.

"Let me give you some examples. I can ask you to relax, but can I make you relax?"

"No," Ed said.

"What if I asked you to close your eyes? Could I force you to do that?" Bob asked.

"No, I don't see how " Ed said.

"What I can do is ask you to do the things that will prepare you and guide you into hypnosis, but you have to do the work," Bob said. "So, with that explanation, you can understand that you put yourself into hypnosis. That simply means all hypnosis is really self-hypnosis, doesn't it?"

"I get it now," Ed said. "I'm driving the car and you're giving me directions, but it's still up to me to turn the wheel."

"Yeah," John said. "That's a good way to look at it."

"To help alleviate your concerns," Bob said, "I'll give you hypnosis scripts you can read to yourselves to induce a trance, make it deeper, suggestions to use, and a process to reawaken you out of trance."

"If we decide we don't like something, we can just re-word it or scratch it out?" Jean asked.

"Yes," Bob said. "You'll have complete editorial control."

"Could you back up for just a second," Ed said. "Can you go into a little more about what you mean by inducing hypnosis?"

"Isn't using the words to 'just imagine,' an induction?" John asked.

"Yes, it is," Bob said. "And we'll use that a lot throughout the sessions. For your purposes, I'd like to use a more formal induction."

"A formal induction does what?" John asked.

"A formal induction does a number of different things," Bob said. "It will help you get focused, give yourself permission to go into trance, prepare you to go to a deeper level of trance, and open your mind to follow acceptable suggestions, first at the conscious level that then at the subconscious level."

"The induction prepares us to go deeper?" Ed asked. "What does that mean?"

"Deepening means that once the induction gets you into a very light state of trance, there is a script you can read to go to a deeper level of trance."

"What happens to us when we go deeper?" Ed asked.

"You gain different capabilities and have different experiences," Bob said. "Think about hypnosis being a continuum from very light to very deep. Let me describe some of the things that happen at the different levels we'll call light, medium, and deep."

"This will be interesting," John said.

"At the light level," Bob said, "your attention and imagination become sufficiently engaged that the sounds and noises around you fade into the background. You're still aware of them, but they're not as intrusive."

"Like a daydream?" Betty asked.

Bob nodded his head and continued.

"With light trance, people are sometimes startled and momentarily disoriented when they are abruptly brought out of trance."

"That happens to me all the time," Jean said. "I'll be focused on something in the boutique and a customer will come in that I didn't hear enter. You should see me jump when they call out to me. I must live in a trance."

"This is usually why some people don't even recognize that they've been in a trance until they come out," Bob said.

"Is that when I know clearly that I'm in trance?" John asked.

"That certainly could be," Bob said. "One way to determine if you were in trance is based on whether you were engaging your imagination and if so, were you responding physically or emotionally to what you imagined."

"So if I was being creative and imagining how I would decorate or layout items, I could be in trance," Jean said. "But if I were doing some task such as threading a needle or calculating profit margins, that most likely would not be trance but rather just intense concentration?"

"I think that's a good way to describe it," Bob said. "When you go into hypnosis as you'll be doing here, you will know you're going into trance and so you'll recognize the signs. It's the unintentional trance that catches you off guard."

Eager to move on, Ed said, "OK, I understand the light stage. What's next?"

"The medium level," Bob said. "When you reach this level you'll know something different is happening. Your breathing will change rhythm by either speeding up or slowing down for a brief time and then continue on deep and slow. You might become sensitive to temperature changes. If we were using relaxation as part of the process, you might lose muscle tone."

"What if I'm not comfortable the way I'm sitting or feel cool? Can I change position or pull a blanket over me without coming out of trance?" Betty asked.

"To some extent, you will need to shift your focused attention away from your imagery and to that degree, you will come up to a lighter state but not completely out of trance, unless you want to come out," Bob said.

"That said, please adjust your position to make yourself more comfortable anytime you do this. Most of the time, you can just continue reading and go right back into a trance. But if you've come up too far, I'll show you a quick trance-induction method you can use to put you back just as deep as you were before."

"OK, so the less we get distracted from what we're doing, the better off we'll be," Ed said.

"Well, you wouldn't want a movie you're watching to be constantly interrupted, would you?" Bob asked.

"No," Ed said. "That would certainly ruin the moment."

"As much as you can, you'll want to find a time and place where you're least likely to be distracted. You'll be using trance a number of times to help you achieve your goals. You can set an alarm clock if you have to do something at a certain time and you're worried you might still be doing one of the trance sessions and not ready to come up and out."

"That will work for me," Betty said.

"One other point while we're talking about it, you don't want to go into trance while you're doing something that requires your full attention like cooking, driving, or caring for infants or children."

"That makes sense," Ed said. "Betty, did you hear that?"

"Yes, Ed," Betty said, rolling her eyes.

"OK," Bob said, "let's take a look at what you might experience at the deep level of hypnosis. By no means is it necessary to go to this level of trance for weight control, but I want you to be aware of some of the things you could experience at this level."

"Good idea," said Jean. "If something strange happened that I wasn't ready for, it would certainly be cause for concern."

"At this deep level, you may feel detached. You may feel a pleasant state of euphoria. You may be very aware of your surroundings but lose any desire to shift position or answer the phone, because to you, at that moment, it might seem like too much trouble. It's as though you'd rather stay and enjoy the moment of this trance state.

"Also," Bob said, "you may experience sensations of lightness and floating or experience sensations of heaviness and sinking into the chair. You might not remember part of the experience."

"Is that like driving home and not remembering the trip?" Ed asked.

"Very much so," Bob said. "You may have been in a light trance overall, but spontaneous memory loss is a characteristic of the deeper levels."

"That's a scary thought," John said.

"Yes, it is," Bob said. "The more you know about hypnosis and how you continuously and spontaneously slip in and out of trance can be pretty important."

"No kidding," Ed said.

"One other characteristic you might want to be aware of that happens at this deeper level trance is analgesia or even complete anesthesia," Bob said. "Experiencing that is not a part of the purpose of what we're trying to accomplish, so we won't intentionally do that. But you should be aware that it could occur spontaneously if you choose to go into this level trance."

"That's what you mentioned for dentists using hypnosis," Ed said.

"At this level, it can happen spontaneously," Bob said. "At the medium level, you could suggest it and get it as well."

"I'll bet that's why some people use hypnosis for natural childbirth," Jean said.

"That and to create a state of deep relaxation, reduce stress, achieve deep sleep, positive outlook, and get a feeling of well-being, among other things," Bob said.

"What happens if I experience anesthesia on part of my body? Will it go away?" Ed asked.

"All the characteristic capabilities of each level of trance will go away as soon as you move up to the next lighter stage unless a specific suggestion has been made and accepted to keep it," Bob said.

"Well, does that mean what we did to achieve our goals will also go away?" Jean asked.

"Not at all," Bob said. "We've been talking about the characteristics or capabilities available at different levels of trance depth. They enhance your ability to communicate with your subconscious mind."

"Like hanging up my phone after I've made a call," John said. "I got the information I wanted but no longer have the means to continue the conversation."

"Exactly," Bob said. "Hypnosis facilitates communication with your subconscious mind, just as your phone does with another person a long distance away."

"I hate to be the one to bring this up," Ed said, "but can we get hurt doing this?"

"Let me be very direct and clear," Bob said. "In all my research, I've not found a single case where someone has been harmed by using hypnosis as you will be doing for weight control purposes."

"I do have another question, and that is if I go into trance, are you sure I won't get stuck and not come out again?" Ed asked.

"This is a very important question and one that everyone needs to be very clear about because unless you feel really comfortable about this," Bob said, "you'll have concerns in the back of your mind, which may prevent you from deliberately putting yourself into a trance."

"I was worried about that as well," Jean said.

"Then let's go ahead and address this now," Bob said. "At the beginning of each of the hypnosis scripts that I give you,

I'll reinforce the fact that if something should happen and you need to be alert, you will be able to come out of trance immediately ready to do what you need to do.

"Further, since you're the person putting yourself into a trance, you'll certainly be able to bring yourself out any time you want. And, at the end of each script, you'll read a particular paragraph letting you know that you won't be able to go back into this level of trance unless you bring yourself out when requested to do so. You'll also read the count from 'one to three' with statements to bring you increasingly to full conscious awareness."

"And if all that doesn't work?" Ed asked.

"I've only come across a couple of instances where the hypnotist just let the person transition to natural sleep," Bob said. "They evidently needed the rest. They didn't stay long and they brought themselves out. But I have never heard or read about a single instance where the person didn't come out of trance."

Everyone nodded their heads in understanding.

"But just to be sure you're comfortable, let's work with a couple of examples," Bob said. "Think about the last movie you watched where you were totally caught up in the story. After the movie, you might have felt a little dazed. Not quite able to think clearly. Thoughts of the movie kept floating in and out of your awareness."

"Yes, I recognize that feeling," Jean said, and everyone agreed.

"You were pretty deep in trance," Bob said. "The movie ended but there was no one guiding you out of trance. You had to find your own way back up to conscious reality, hopefully before you started driving anywhere."

"Now it makes more sense," Ed said. "I've never been stuck in trance in a movie, but I've watched a couple of them where it took a long time before I could concentrate on anything else."

"Had you told yourself that you would come immediately awake if something required your attention," Bob said, "you could bring yourself out of trance faster. But then again, before our conversation, you weren't aware that those experiences were trances."

"Now I'm much more comfortable with the whole idea of trance," Ed said. "When I run into something as new to me as hypnosis, I really need to fully explore it before I can embrace it. But I'm totally on board now."

Bob took a deep breath and said, "Hypnosis is the quickest, easiest, and most effective way to communicate directly with your subconscious mind so it knows exactly what you want to do with the size and shape of your body.

"You can drastically reduce the fattening and other ill-effects of stress by using effective coping strategies both with and without going into a formally induced trance.

"Through hypnosis, you will be able to find and power up motivators operating at the subconscious level to help you through the rough spots.

"It will help you find and change hidden blocker beliefs and turn them into supportive beliefs.

"Hypnosis will help you harness the power of the fear center so that it reacts to help you keep rather than stopping you from getting the body you want.

"And finally, there will be times when you run into a challenge where you need to call up some of your internal resources such as passion or courage or some other personal capability so that you to see it successfully through," Bob said. "Hypnosis is a great way to identify and energize these resources."

"Is that all?" Ed asked.

Incredulous looks and then laughter at Ed's dry wit. It does come in handy.

"This has been a really good discussion," Bob said. "If you want to use hypnosis to help you achieve your weight, size, and shape goals, I'll be happy to guide you through the process."

Heads nodded enthusiastically.

"We're ready," John said. "When can we get started?"

"How about tomorrow," Bob said.

"Anything we need to do?" Jean asked.

"Yes," Bob said. "Find out what your weight range should be and see if you have any photos of yourselves when you were at that weight."

"Anything else?" Betty asked.

"That's all that we need for our next session," Bob said. "I'll bring copies of the hypnosis scripts' and we'll take some time to go into trance and experience first-hand what we've been talking about."

"Same time tomorrow?" Betty asked.

Heads nodded. Growing expectations and anticipation of going into trance were high on everyone's mind.

Chapter 4 Create Your New Body Image

After gathering back at Ed and Betty's condo, Bob asked, "Did everyone get to look up their recommended weight ranges for your height and bone structure?"

"Yes," Betty said. "We were talking about that just before you got here."

"We were shocked when we saw the low numbers in the ranges presented," Jean said.

"Over the years, I guess we've really developed a warped sense of what our weight should be," John said.

"That got Betty and me to start thinking about portion size," Ed said. "We discovered that what we thought were normal portions and what were actually normal portions was so far out of whack, we had to get out Betty's measuring cups and rethink what's normal."

"Yeah," Jean said. "We were so far over the top in our super-sized thinking, we had to recalibrate back to a normal world with normal-size people eating normal size portions."

"What about body size and shape?" Bob asked.

"We started to look for some old pictures of when we used to be that size," John said. "I told Jean that the last time I was anywhere near that size was my senior year when I was on the skiing team. Unfortunately, most of my photos show me in full gear, but I still look really fit."

"That's when we decided to look through catalogs and magazines to cut out pictures of people wearing the clothes and swimsuits we'd like to wear close to the sizes we'd like to be," Jean said. "That gave us a much a better idea of what we should look like without our excess fat. It really helped."

Betty said, "I've always been heavy. I come from a family of big eaters, and I love to cook, so I'm really in a bind. I'll need to do what Jean and John are doing and go get my catalogs."

"I found some pictures when I weighed about what I want to get to and I was pretty athletic and still have a good amount of muscle that I don't want to lose along with the fat," Ed said. "We talked about this before and we're really talking about using hypnosis to reduce excess fat and fat alone, aren't we?"

"Correct," Bob said. "Fat is the target. You'll need to keep your muscle to tone and sculpt your body."

"That'll work," Ed said.

"If you want your subconscious mind to help you achieve your ideal weight, size, and shape," Bob said, "you have to help it know exactly what that is using as many of your physical senses and your emotions as you can."

"I could use some body sculpting for sure," Jean said.

"Jean," John said, "sculpting also means muscle tone and that means the 'E' word. That's 'E' for 'exercise.'"

"Ugh, I know," Jean said.

"Remember the story about how Michelangelo created his sculptures?" Bob asked.

"What do you mean?" Ed asked.

"There is a story about how Michelangelo was once asked how he could create such a beautiful statue from a block of marble," Bob said. "He replied that first, he saw the statue inside the block of marble in great detail. And then he said that all he did was to remove the excess marble from around it so that everyone else could see it as well."

"I get it," Ed said. "Our fat is our marble and right now we're both the statue and the sculptor"

"What we've got to do first is to see what we look like without all this extra fat," John said.

"Exactly," Bob said. "To help you get there, I'm going to take you through an imagery process where I will guide you to think about different parts of your body and then change them to their ideal size and shape so your subconscious mind will have a very clear picture of what you want it to create."

"This is how we replace the body image our subconscious mind has of us now," John said.

"That's right," Bob said. "For example, you'll focus on your face, imagine removing the fat, imagine increasing the muscle tone to add more shape and definition and then imagine what that end result looks like. And then, you'll simply continue down with each of the major body part groupings, changing them to your desired size and shape. This is what's called body sculpting and is an exceptionally effective hypnosis technique.

"You'll want to do this process at least three or four times over the next few days until the image you have in your mind is clear, consistent, and easily imagined, to the point where you could just think about it and have it instantly appear in front of you. You'll know you're there when the details in your imagery become life like."

"Will we be going into a hypnotic trance when we do this?" Ed asked.

"Yes," Bob said. "You'll use this body sculpting imagery during the deepening process. As we read the trance induction and the deepening scripts, I'll guide you with the suggested imagery and then I'll guide you as you read the reawakening to bring you out of trance."

"This is what we talked about earlier where we go to a deeper level of trance?" Ed asked.

"Yes," Bob said. "To do this I usually like to count down from 10 to 1, using a staircase that you can walk or float down."

Create Your New Body Image

"Why down?" Ed asked. "Is there some significance to going down?"

"Just a little," Bob said. "Going to a deeper level of trance is usually associated with the direction down. For many people, it's easier to conceptualize going 'down deeper' than going 'up deeper.' But, 'coming up' is a term we'll use to come back up to conscious level and out of trance."

"Got it," Ed said.

"Can we take a quick break," Betty asked. "We've been sitting here for a while, and I don't want to miss anything if I have to step out."

"Absolutely," Bob said. "Good idea."

After a short break, Bob passed around copies of the first hypnosis script and asked, "Are you ready to go into hypnosis?"

All heads nodded.

"We'll start with a version of the ever popular 'BLINK' trance induction," Bob said. "It's quick and easy, and it'll take you right into a light hypnotic state where we can then deepen it so you can work with the suggestions. Every time you do this, you'll train your brain to go quicker and deeper into a trance so you can easily get to a depth where you feel comfortable and effective."

"What if I have questions while we're in hypnosis?" Jean asked.

"From time-to-time, I'll pause so that we can discuss what is happening in your experience. Since I won't formally bring you out of trance for these discussions, you'll stay mostly in a trance while we talk. It will be similar to the dazed feeling Ed talked about after being deeply in trance during a great movie."

"I'm worried I might come out completely," Betty said.

"And you might, but that's OK. I'll do the short version of the induction after we talk so that you can slide right back in as deep as before. In fact, most of the time, you may go a little deeper. Going in and out of trance is actually a very effective deepening technique."

"I'd like that," Betty said.

"OK," Bob said, "ready?"

Everyone confirmed they were ready.

Bob said, "And if it meets with your approval, will you do what I ask you to do?"

"Yes," they said in unison while nodding their heads.

"Good," Bob said. "Always know that if anything happens that requires your attention while you're in hypnosis, you'll be able to come up and out immediately, fully alert and ready to deal with it.

"Let's start by releasing some of the muscle tension and mental distractions by taking a deep breath and as you exhale feel the tension flow out of your body.

"Again, take a deep refreshing and cleansing breath and exhale. Continue to breathe deeply and comfortably for a little while longer. Focus on your breathing.

"Should you become aware of any sounds or other distractions, simply notice them, let them increase your focus and concentration on this process, and then let them fade away into the background.

"When you read the word 'Breathe' on your hypnosis script, take a deep breath, exhale and continue reading.

"Take your time with this.

"Whenever you read the word 'BLINK' on your hypnosis script, please blink your eyes and then continue reading.

"Here we go. Want it to happen, expect it to happen, allow it to happen.

"Breathe.

"Five, BLINK.

"Feeling good, focused, anticipating going into trance.

"BLINK.
"No pressure, no rush, slow down.
"BLINK.
"Breathe deeply and exhale. Focus on your breathing.
"Four, BLINK.
"Slowing down.
"BLINK.
"Open to the experience.
"BLINK.
"Going down, deeper down.
"Three, BLINK.
"BLINK.
"Focus on your breathing while you read.
"BLINK.
"Breathe deeply and exhale.
"Going slower now.
"Two, BLINK.
"Wonderful feeling going deeper and deeper into trance.
"BLINK.
"Narrow your focus to what you're reading.
"BLINK.
"Breathe deeply and exhale. In, out, in, out.
"Slower and deeper down.
"One, BLINK.
"Drifting down, feeling good.
"BLINK.
"Focus on the words you're reading, and let the background fade away.
"BLINK.
"Going deeper, deeper down.
"You can blink normally and automatically now.
"Breathe deeply and exhale.

"Whenever you're in trance at any level, you will always be able to read my words to continue through the session and reawaken out of trance when it's time to do so.

"Now that you're comfortable, let's start making sure the image of what you want your body to look like is clear and imprinted on your subconscious mind.

"Imagine that you're at the top of a 10-step staircase.

"At the bottom of your staircase is a room where you can communicate directly with your subconscious mind.

"Imagine now that you're looking down at the staircase. Are the steps made of marble, wood, or are they carpeted? Is the staircase wide and grand or more narrow and bright?

"What about the handrail? Where is it placed? What is it made of? What shape does it take?

"It's your staircase and handrail and so you can make them as you wish.

"Each time you go down a step, you'll notice your concentration increase and your focus narrow as you drift deeper and deeper into trance. You can either step down or gently float down the stairs.

"If you're ready now, let's start down the staircase one step at a time.

"Ten. Hold the handrail and notice its texture and temperature. Take a deep breath and as you exhale, go down a step.

"Nine. Focus on your face. Imagine how you want it to look that's different than it is now. Look closely at your forehead, eyes, cheeks, and chin.

"Notice the change when you remove excess fat and tighten the skin. Mentally exercise the muscles in your face. Notice how they give your face a lift.

"Take a deep breath, and as you exhale, go down a step.

"Eight. Imagine and narrow your focus to your jaw and neck. How would you want them to change as you remove the excess fat and tighten the skin?

"Imagine them slim and trim.

"Mentally exercise and tone the muscles in your neck and jaw to create the physical appearance that is natural and attractive for your bone structure. See the change now.

"Take a deep breath, and as you exhale, go down a step.

"Seven. Imagine and focus on your shoulders and back.

"Imagine removing any excess fat and changing them to your desired slim and trim size and shape.

"Mentally exercise the muscles in your shoulders and back. Feel the muscle tone under your skin. Imagine what that looks like. See the change now.

"In a moment, we're going to pause and talk about what you're experiencing. You can stay in trance while we do this. Stay in trance.

"John, what are you experiencing that's working for you?" Bob asked.

"I never really thought about how my face would look without the excess fat," he said.

"Jean, what about you?" Bob asked.

"I was amazed at the muscles in my face that I could exercise," she said. "It was like you said, I was getting a facelift. I don't like exercise, but I think I could get to like it a lot if it works the way I think it's going to."

"Betty, how has this been so far for you?" Bob asked.

"I just stared at the hypnosis scripts you gave us and when you said blink," she said, "I saw the word blink and then I blinked. Mostly I just followed along. Sometimes I think I imagined reading it. When we started down the staircase, I couldn't believe how clear it was. I can describe it in every detail."

"Somehow I've got a feeling you will," Bob said.

"Ed, how about you? What are you experiencing?"

"I'm not sure how well I'm doing. I mean, I saw the staircase, but it seems more of a distant thought than something real," he said.

"Just being able to imagine the staircase is the first clue that you're probably in or about to go into at least a very light trance level," Bob said. "With that as a start, after you do this a few times, you'll soon be going deeper and deeper until you reach the level where you feel the most comfortable to accomplish your goals.

"Very good … Breathe …

"In a moment, you will count backward from three to one using the 'BLINK' method. Each time you read the word 'BLINK,' please blink and each time you blink, you will go back into hypnosis at a deeper level than before.

"Want it to happen, expect it to happen, and let it happen.

"Three. BLINK.

"Focus on the words you're reading, and let the background fade away.

"Breathe.

"Two. BLINK.

"Feeling good, going deeper into trance.

"Breathe.

"One. BLINK.

"Going down, deeper down.

"Blink normally and automatically.

"Good, you're doing fine. Let's continue down the staircase.

"Take a deep breath, and as you exhale, go down a step.

"Six. Imagine and focus on your arms, elbows, forearms, hands, and fingers.

"Imagine removing the excess fat and loose skin, allowing them to change to your desired slim and trim size and shape.

"Mentally exercise and tone the muscles in your arms and hands to create the physical appearance that is natural and attractive for you. See the change now.

"Take a deep breath, and as you exhale, go down a step.

"Five. Imagine and focus on your chest.

"Notice how it gently moves each time you breathe.

"Breathe.

"And as your chest moves, imagine it changing to your desired size and shape.

"Mentally exercise and tone the muscles in your chest to create the physical appearance that is natural and attractive for you. See it change now.

"Take a deep breath, and as you exhale, go down a step.

"Four. Focus now on your stomach area, waist, and lower back.

"Imagine removing the excess fat around your stomach area, waist, and lower back and seeing the change to your desired slim and trim size and shape.

"See your waist exactly as you want it. View it from the front, from the side, from the back.

"Mentally exercise and tone the muscles in your stomach area, waist, and lower back to create the physical appearance that is natural and attractive for you. See the change now.

"Take a deep breath, and as you exhale, go down a step.

"Three. Imagine and focus on your hips.

"Imagine removing the excess fat and seeing them change to your desired slim and trim size and shape.

"Mentally exercise and tone the muscles around your hips to create the physical appearance that is natural and attractive for you. See the change now.

"Stay in trance while we talk for a moment about what you are experiencing.

"Breathe.

"Ed, what are you experiencing now?" Bob asked.

Sounding more lethargic than before, he said, "I'm finding muscles I didn't know I had."

"Betty, what about you?"

"It was really hard to imagine the whole area around my stomach changing. I'm having trouble imagining what that will look like. I need to go back and do that again until I can."

"Jean?"

"I know what Betty's saying," Jean said. "I was really having to focus extra hard for this. I had to remember one of the pictures we cut out to even get that image in my mind and then I had to imagine the fat melting away."

"John?"

"When I'm mentally exercising muscles, I sometimes noticed that I was actually making slight physical movements. This is making me much more aware of my body," he said.

Jean looked at John and said, "I feel the same way. It's as though I'm discovering myself all over again."

"Good," Bob said. "We're all on target and doing fine.

"In a moment, I'll count backward again from three to one using an abbreviated version of the 'BLINK' re-induction method.

"While I'm doing that, look at your hypnosis scripts and each time you read 'BLINK,' please blink and that will help you go back into a deeper state of hypnosis than before.

"Want it to happen, watch it happen, let it happen.

"Three, blink, blink, blink, down, down, down.

"Two, blink, blink, deeper and deeper.

"One, blink, down deeper.

"Blinking normally now.

Create Your New Body Image

"Breathe ...

"Good, you're doing fine ...

"And now continuing down the staircase ...

"Take a deep breath, and as you exhale, go down a step.

"Two. Imagine and focus on your legs.

"Imagine removing all the excess fat and seeing them change to your desired slim and trim size and shape.

"See them from the front, from the side, from the back.

"Mentally exercise and tone the muscles in your legs. See and feel the muscle tone under your skin. Imagine creating the physical appearance that is natural and attractive for you. See the change now.

"Take a deep breath, and as you exhale, go down a step.

"One. Imagine and focus on your ankles, feet, and toes.

"Imagine removing any excess fat and then seeing them change to your desired slim and trim size and shape.

"Look down at your ankles and feet. Imagine them as you want them to look and feel. In your mind, stretch and move your toes. Feel good.

"Mentally exercise and tone the muscles in your ankles, feet, and toes to create the physical appearance that is natural and attractive for you. See the change now.

"Holding on to the handrail, take a deep breath, exhale, and go down into the room at the bottom of the staircase.

"In this very special room, you are communicating your thoughts, feelings, and images directly to your subconscious mind and it is sensing, watching, and learning.

"Look around the room, and notice at one end, there us a set of full-length mirrors positioned at angles so that when you try on clothes, you can see yourself from the front, sides, and back.

"These are very special mirrors in that they can only reflect what the subconscious mind believes to be real. When the mirrors reflect what you imagine, then the subconscious mind is letting you know that it understands and believes the imagined you is real. This is the body it will now guide you to make in your physical reality.

"Next to the mirrors is an open closet filled with clothes, from swimsuits to formal wear, in the size you want. You can instantly change clothes and you can add or remove clothes as you wish.

"At the other end of the room, there is a tall table with a book and a pen on it, and in the middle, between the mirrors and the desk, there is a large door.

"This room is of your own creation so make it as comfortable, private, and safe for you as you would like it to be. Put your own colors on the walls, add throw rugs or carpet, put trim on the mirrors, and stock your closet with the clothes you want in the sizes you want.

"For now, you will work with the mirrors to make sure your subconscious mind can clearly see and believe this is the real body you want.

"Select from your open closet the clothes you want to wear in the size you want. Instantly put them on. Notice how easily they go on and how good they fit your slim, trim, physically fit body.

"With your new clothes on, imagine with all your senses what it feels like to look good in them. Feel those clothes on your body. Smell how fresh they are. Hear the movement of the material.

"Feel yourself moving in them. Sense how comfortable they feel all over your body.

"Now imagine standing in front of the mirrors in your room so you can view your physical image from the front, from the side, and from the back wearing your favorite clothes.

Create Your New Body Image

"Realize that the muscle tone you've achieved helps make these clothes look so good.

"Notice the improvements in your posture and how much better that makes the clothes look on you.

"You believe this slim and trim person is the true you. Hold that image in your mind with all your senses actively involved. Say to yourself, 'I believe this slim and trim person is the true me. I believe this is my real body.

"Make sure your subconscious mind is clear on what you want and that this is your true body. Look carefully at the image. Is this the body you want being reflected in the mirrors? What you see is what your subconscious mind understands and believes you want.

"Take a moment now and ask your subconscious mind to let you know when it believes that this is your true physical size and shape that it is to guide you to make in your physical reality.

"Wait for a shift or feeling of some sort acknowledging the subconscious mind is adopting your image as its own. It could happen now or in just a moment.

"Ask your subconscious mind to guide you during your daily life about what you must do to help create the body it now believes is the true you.

"You're doing fine. Breathe

"Become aware and be open to the guidance your subconscious mind provides.

"You are slim, trim, and physically fit so act and eat like the slim, trim, physically fit person you believe yourself to be.

"Hear yourself say, "I am slim, trim, and physically fit, with good muscle tone at a size and shape that is right and attractive for my body's height and frame. I think, act, and eat like the slim, trim, physically fit person I am.

"You're doing fine. Take a deep breath and let it out.

"Say silently to yourself. 'I believe this is my true size and shape. It is me. I own it. I'm grateful that my subconscious mind can learn and do everything in its power to quickly, automatically, and safely make this the real physical me.'

"Good, you're doing fine. Breathe.

"It's time now to go to the staircase, reach out, and hold the handrail.

"Notice how comfortably deep in trance you've become. Each time you read yourself into hypnosis, you will find it easier and easier to go into a deeper level of trance so that you quickly achieve the level that is right for you to communicate effectively with your subconscious mind.

"And now, ready.

"Go up to step one in your slim, trim, physically fit body. It's yours now and forever.

"Go up to step two. Feel grateful that your subconscious mind understands and believes in what you want and is now taking action to bring it to physical reality.

"Go up to step three. Notice how your feet, legs, and hips look and move as you go up the stairs.

"Go up to step four. Observe your stomach, waist, lower back. Watch your muscles moving.

"Go up to step five. See your chest moving as you breathe. It's just as you want it to be.

"Go up to step six. Notice your hand on the handrail. Watch your arms move.

"Go up to step seven. See your shoulders and back, muscles toned and moving smoothly.

"Go up to step eight. Observe your jaw and neck. See how they look. They are just as you want them to be.

"Go up to step nine. Notice the smile on your slim, trim face.

"Go up to step ten. Now mentally step back into your body and feel wonderful about the experiences you're having.

"Good, you're doing fine. Breathe.

"You've done well. In a moment, I will count you up and out of trance.

"If you want to intentionally go back to this level of trance in the future, you must agree to bring yourself out of trance when asked to do so.

"Let's start to count up so that you can easily bring yourself up and back into the present time and place.

"One. Coming up now, take a deep breath and come up now.

"Two. Begin to move your body, stretch, and come up even more now.

"Three. Wide awake and back in the present, feeling refreshed, alert, and fully awake.

"Just stay where you are for a moment while you increase your alertness. Stretch a little and adjust your posture to help become fully alert."

Bob paused for a minute and then asked, "How was that?"

"Wow," Jean said.

"Me, too," Betty said. "The staircase and room were so real. Now I know what Alice experienced going down the rabbit hole.

"I'm not sure how much of this I read as you were guiding us," John said, "but I was definitely feeling that something very different was going on with me."

Ed looked a little perplexed and asked, "Even though I was totally engaged, there were times when I was aware of some of the things going on around me, so was I in trance or not?"

"At the light level of trance, you would notice things going on around you," Bob said. "Were there times when those things seemed to fade into the background?"

"Almost every time you said to 'imagine' something like my face or arm, I was able to focus and concentrate on seeing and feeling it in its reshaped size."

"What about the 'BLINK' induction? How did that work for you?"

"About the third or fourth 'BLINK,' I knew something was happening, but I guess I was trying too hard to understand what was happening rather than just let it happen."

"What about when we stopped to talk about what you were experiencing? Do you think you came completely out or almost out or pretty much stayed in trance?"

"I think I came pretty far out because I wanted to hear what was being said."

"From what you're telling me," Bob said, "I think you actually went a little deeper than the very light level you were in before. Congratulations, first time taking the guided tour and you did just fine."

John said, "At first, I was in a daze and wasn't sure who was talking until you called my name. And then I think I came all the way out."

"What happened after you answered?" Bob asked.

"I don't know," John said. "It seems like I was just sitting here sort of numb, but not. Do you know what I mean?"

"That's very common to slide right back into trance with your mind blank. That's one of the reasons to count yourself up and out of trance each time you intentionally put yourself into hypnosis. Take a little time to get fully alert. Get up and move around."

"John looked zoned out when I looked at him," Jean said and then asked, "Were we talking funny?"

"I didn't notice anyone's voices dragging too much as would normally occur at a deep level trance," Bob said. "But I did notice your facial expressions go blank along with that

Create Your New Body Image

intense stare as you read your hypnosis scripts along with me. That tells me your visual imagery was in overdrive."

"That's a good look, I'm sure," Jean said.

"What about when we talked to you? Did we keep the same zoned out look?" Ed asked.

"Sometimes more and sometimes less," Bob said. "When you go into trance, you don't stay at one level all the time. You move up and down."

"I have another question," Betty said. "When Ed and I do this by ourselves, is it necessary to always talk about it as we go through it like we did here?"

"Not at all," Bob said. You can do the entire process by yourself or with Ed and not talk about it during the time you're in trance."

"What about the 'three, two, one, BLINK' re-induction you had us use to return to trance? If we don't really come all the way out, do we need to do that each time?" John asked.

"No you don't," Bob said. "After you've done this a few times, the cues to send you back into trance will begin to work automatically. It may be the word 'imagine' or some other word or cue that takes you back in. Just always be sure you want to go into trance and at the end always bring yourself out."

"Oh, yeah I can see it now," Ed said. "I'm in the conference room and my boss says, 'just imagine' and out I go."

"Those are the magic words, aren't they?" John said.

"That's a good reason for learning the ins and outs about hypnosis," Bob said. "This knowledge and experience can keep you from unintentionally sliding in or at least knowing that's what's happening. Always consciously agree to go into hypnosis, and if you don't agree, you can quickly bring yourself out of trance."

"One quick question," Betty said. "On the hypnosis scripts you gave us, how closely should we follow the wording? Do we need to use the exact same words you used?"

"You can be close and it will work," Bob said. "For example, on the BLINK re-induction to trance, you could change up the words to something like, 'Three. BLINK, going down now. Two. BLINK, deeper down now. One. BLINK, breathe and imagine.' Or you could just say, 'three, two, one, going down, deeper down,' then focus your imagination and you're back in."

"That's good to know," John said. "When we come out of trance to talk about something we're experiencing, all we have to do then is the 'three, two, one' imagine routine and we're back in?"

"Yes," Bob said.

"Do we have to count ourselves up each time we come out to talk?" Jean asked.

"No, don't do that," Bob said. "Only count yourself up and out of trance at the very end."

"Since this is all eyes open once we know how to do it, can we just close our eyes after the last BLINK and do it before we go to sleep?" Jean asked.

"Sure," Bob said. "That's a very good way to do it. Even then, if you're in bed ready to drift off to sleep, you don't have to count yourself back up to into full alertness. It would be good at step three to say something like, 'Three. Drifting off now into a deep natural sleep.' Remember different parts of the brain are active when you're in hypnosis than when you're in natural sleep."

"Hey, I know," Jean said. "Can I just close my eyes while John reads this to me?"

"Certainly," Bob said. "You might take turns guiding each other."

Create Your New Body Image

"Can we do this anywhere?" Betty asked.

"Yes," Bob said. "But even though you're doing it with your eyes open, don't ask Ed to read it to you while you're driving.

"For that matter, like I mentioned before, don't do any deliberate trance work while you're doing anything that requires your full attention like cooking, driving, or watching over children. We really have to be careful because sometimes what we're doing is so boring we can find ourselves in tranceland before we know it."

"Hear that, Betty?" Ed asked, expecting the eye roll once again.

Ignoring him she asked, "What's behind the door and why do we have a book and pen?"

"You'll find out in later sessions," Bob said. "Right now they're being used as props to build anticipation to help you go into trance quickly."

"I had so much fun picking clothes off the rack and trying them on," Betty said. "I must have tried on three different outfits. I like that instant change routine."

Jean asked, "When I asked my subconscious mind to let me know when it believed that this was my true body to let me know, I felt a jolt. It was a physical jolt. Is that normal?"

"There is a wide range of things that happen from a simple warm feeling of understanding or a deeper calmness all the way to the kind of jolt you had," Bob said. "Any of the signs let you know you're having an impact on your subconscious mind."

"I didn't have any of these happen," Ed said. "Betty, did you?"

"I had a peaceful feeling that felt like acceptance," she said.

"But nothing like a jolt?"

"No."

"Hmm," Ed said. "I'd rather it to be a dramatic sign like Jean got, but I'll take what I can get. Maybe it happened and I just wasn't aware."

"It could be anywhere from very subtle to dramatic," Bob said. "You'll learn to become more sensitive and aware of them as you continue to use what you've learned and will learn in our upcoming sessions."

"Do you think my doubts about this process or being able to get my body the way I want has anything to do with it?" Ed asked.

"I think so," Bob said. "If you don't believe it's possible when you're communicating with your subconscious mind, there's no way that I know of that it will believe something you don't."

"What do I do then?" Ed asked.

"If you don't have a clear and strong belief in the process," Bob said, "you really should suspend disbelief until it proves out one way or the other. Give it the benefit of the doubt. Go with it as far as you can."

"I can get part of the way there," Ed said. "I've had some good experiences here with everyone. It just seems like such a huge leap for me."

"When we take a three- or four-day driving trip," Jean said, "we have to set our goals for each day or it would make us crazy thinking about how much farther we had to go."

"But you still have your ultimate destination in mind," Bob said.

"Well, yes," Jean said.

"Setting milestone goals is also a good way to keep from getting discouraged," Bob said. "Just so long as you don't lose sight of your ultimate goal."

"If I can set intermediate goals," Ed said, "then I think I'm OK."

"Yes, of course," Bob said. "But again there is one condition. You keep your ultimate goal of getting the body you want in the back of your mind at all times and use that imagery when you're working in trance. Agreed?"

Ed nodded.

"Is there a quick way to tell if our ultimate goal was accepted by the subconscious mind?" Betty asked.

"Yes," Bob said. "The first test is to close your eyes and ask, 'what does my body look like?' You should immediately see the body you imagined. If not, ask, 'what does the body I want look like?' Now if you have a big difference, you'll need to do more trance work to convince your subconscious mind that the body it imagines and the body you want are the same."

"I just did that and I'm going to need more trance work," Betty said.

"We'll be doing more activities in trance that will help add clarity to your body image. It really is important for your subconscious mind to know what it's supposed to be doing for you."

"By the way, does anyone have an idea about how much time has passed since we started our session this evening?" Bob asked.

"Oh my," Betty said. "I had no idea."

"This should let you know that you've been deeply engaged in this conversation and the trance experience, which led to some time distortion, which is a characteristic of a light trance," Bob said.

"I'm usually very good about knowing the time," Ed said. "But this time, I lost all sense of time. That's so unlike me. OK, I'm convinced."

"Why don't we get together again in a few days," Bob said. "I want to give you enough time to go into trance a few more times on your own to create and clarify the imagery your subconscious mind needs to do its job. Be sure to take the copies of the script with you."

Betty said, "OK, I'll coordinate everyone's schedules.

Chapter 5 **Reinforce Your New Body Image**

By the time Jean and John arrived home it was getting late, but they decided to push on and practice the imagery process they had just completed with Dr. Bob.

"This has been fabulous for me," Jean said. "I think it really takes us way down the road to achieving our goals. How'd it work for you?"

"I never thought we'd get this far this fast," John said. "I'm feeling much more confident."

"Me, too," she said. "I'm trying to apply what we learned to what I already know to help make connections and give me more confidence in the process as well."

"That makes sense," he said. "But when we talk about our size and shape goals, I'm not sure I can imagine myself as a skinny person."

"Well, let's not get that carried away," she said. "Skinny may be a little further than we want to go. I think we should focus on becoming slim and trim with good muscle tone so we're not just thin and flabby, but we'll have shape as well."

"But I still can't imagine myself as thin," he said. "I had a real challenge when I was trying to see my goal size and shape earlier in the mirrors. My current shape kept showing up. So I guess that's what my subconscious mind still believes I should look like."

"Let's use our travel strategy like we talked about earlier and just imagine our body changes in smaller steps that we can accept and believe are possible to achieve," she said.

"And then we can recalibrate each time we do take some fat off," he said.

"Yes," she said. "We'll have a new starting point and maybe a new end size and shape as well."

"I think I can do that," he said. "If not, I'm going to try to force the issue."

"What do you mean?" she asked.

"Just that," he said. "I'm going to focus and concentrate so hard on whatever part of my body is not cooperating and just force it into the shape I want."

"Using what?" she asked.

"Why my imagination, of course," he said smiling.

"Let's get our hypnosis scripts out to guide us," she said.

"Yeah," he said, "it seems that if we need our subconscious involved, we need to be in trance."

"OK," she said, "Even after what we just talked about, for tonight, I'm interested in focusing on really making sure I can visualize and fully imagine the end result of what I want my subconscious to go to work on creating for me."

"I'll go as far as I can in imagining my size and shape to be as slim and trim as possible," he said.

"Fair enough," she said. "And remember, we can always pop out of trance wide awake and fully alert if something comes up that needs our full attention. How's that for a quick paraphrase?"

"And now," he said as he continued to read out loud, "let's start by releasing some of the muscle tension and mental distractions by taking a deep breath, and as you exhale, feel the tension flow out of your body.

"Again, take a deep refreshing and cleansing breath and exhale. Continue to breathe deeply and comfortably for a little while longer. Focus on your breathing.

"Should you become aware of any sounds or other distractions, simply notice them, let them increase your focus

Reinforce Your New Body Image

and concentration on this process, and then let them fade away into the background.

"When you read the word 'Breathe' on your hypnosis script, take a deep breath, exhale, and continue reading.

"Take your time with this.

"Whenever you read the word 'BLINK' on your hypnosis script, please blink your eyes and then continue reading.

"Here we go. Want it to happen, expect it to happen, allow it to happen.

John and Jean continued to slowly read the induction silently. Their breathing kept them in sync with each other.

"Breathe.

"Five, BLINK.

"Feeling good, focused, anticipating going into trance.

"BLINK.

"No pressure, no rush, slow down.

"BLINK.

"Breathe deeply and exhale. Focus on your breathing.

"Four, BLINK.

"Slowing down

"BLINK.

"Open to the experience.

"BLINK.

"Going down, deeper down.

"Three, BLINK.

"BLINK.

"Focus on your breathing while you read.

"BLINK.

"Breathe deeply and exhale. In, out, in, out.

"Going slower now.

"Two, BLINK.

"Wonderful feeling going deeper and deeper into trance.

"BLINK.

"Narrow your focus to what you're reading.
"BLINK.
"Breathe deeply and exhale.
"Slower and deeper down.
"One, BLINK.
"Drifting down, feeling good.
"BLINK.
"Focus on the words you're reading, and let the background fade away.
"BLINK.
"Going deeper, deeper down.
"You can blink normally and automatically now.
"Breathe deeply and exhale.
"Whenever you're in trance at any level, you will always be able to read my words to continue through the session and reawaken out of trance when it's time to do so.

Jean and John paused for a moment and then Jean said, "Let's just stay in trance and talk this through, OK?" she asked. "Since I have the script ready for this next part, I'll be the guide for the 10-step staircase."

"Works for me," John said.

"Ten. Hold the handrail and notice its texture and temperature. Take a deep breath and as you exhale, go down a step.

"Nine. Focus on your face. Imagine how you want it to look that's different than it is now. Look closely at your forehead, eyes, cheeks, and chin.

"Notice the change when you remove excess fat and tighten the skin. Mentally exercise the muscles in your face. Notice how they give your face a lift.

Jean spoke first and said, "I'm imagining removing all the excess fat, letting it dissolve and melt away, and now I'm toning and shaping my muscles."

Reinforce Your New Body Image

And then she asked, "John, what do you want your face to look like?"

"What, oh, like I said, I never really thought about that until earlier today."

"While we're here working together on this, why don't you try to get a clearer image of it now?" she asked.

"Yeah, well," he said, "I'd like to get rid of the bags under my eyes, I'd like to reduce my chubby cheeks so they don't bounce when I talk, I'd like to get rid of my jowls, and I'd like to tighten the skin under my chin and around my neck."

"That's a tall order," she said.

"Well, you asked," he said.

"What about you?" he asked.

"Seems we both have a lot of the same areas to tone up," she said.

"In order to tone these areas of our faces," he said, "we discovered that there are real muscles there. Let's see if we can find and tense these muscles. Instead of mentally tensing them, this time I'm going to slightly tense them physically, just enough to notice them."

"Let me try that right now to get a feel for what that would be like," Jean said and then continued, "I'm gently tensing the muscles and now I'm imagining my face relaxing and changing to a slim and trim face. I'm imagining my forehead, cheeks, and chin automatically changing."

"I want to do this one again," she said. "I want to take a little more time with my face since I haven't done this before today. I'm fascinated that I'm going to give myself a facelift that will also recondition my skin."

"OK, me, too," John said. "Eyes closed, just imagining?"

"Yeah," she said. "Let's do that."

After a few moments with their eyes closed, John opened his and said, "I'll bet we can find books on face muscle exercises to help us with this."

"I'd like that," she said.

"Let's move on then," he said. "Take a deep breath, and as you exhale, go down a step.

"Eight. Imagine and narrow your focus to your jaw and neck. How would you want them to change as you remove the excess fat and tighten the skin?

"Imagine them slim and trim.

"Gently exercise the muscles around your jaw and neck. Imagine feeling the skin tightening under your jaw and around your neck to create the physical appearance that is natural and attractive for your bone structure. See the change now."

Jean paused for a moment so they could both image how that looked and felt.

"How did you do with that one?" she asked.

"I really had a hard time with the area under my chin in the jaw area until I pushed my head and jaw forward and then tilted my head back," he said. "That's when I felt my skin and muscles tighten. That means I can exercise that area."

"Interestingly, I pulled on my neck muscles and felt that I could do something about this area too," she said. "OK, let's keep going."

"I'm ready," he said.

"Take a deep breath, and as you exhale, go down a step.

"Seven. Imagine and focus on your shoulders and back.

"Imagine removing any excess fat and changing them to your desired slim and trim size and shape.

"Gently tense and then relax the muscles in shoulders and back. Feel the muscle tone under your skin. Imagine what that looks like. See the change now."

Reinforce Your New Body Image

After a few moments, John said, "I also noticed that when I relaxed that area, I could really tell the difference. I'm holding a lot of tension there."

"So maybe a part of our problem is coming from stress." she said.

"From what I've read in what seem like a thousand articles and from what Dr. Bob said, the tension from the stress we have not only made us miserable but also causes a lot of our belly fat," he said.

"We need to pay more attention to that," she said. "Let's bring that up the next time we're together. For now though, let's keep moving down our bodies, relaxing and imagining."

"Ready to move on to our arms?" she asked.

"Sure."

"OK, back to the staircase," she said. "Take a deep breath, and as you exhale, go down a step.

"Six. Imagine and focus on your arms, elbows, forearms, hands, and fingers.

"Imagine removing the excess fat and loose skin, allowing them to change to your desired slim and trim size and shape."

Jean paused and then said, "I'm going to gently tense and relax each of these muscles in my arms and then close my eyes so I can better imagine them changing to the size and shape I want. I need some time here, so I'll let you know when I'm through with this one."

When Jean finished and opened her eyes she noticed John was looking at her with a pleasant smile on his face and said, "Ready to talk?"

"I am now," she said. "The place that got me is that my skin jiggles under my upper arm, especially when I wave to someone."

"Sounds like your triceps need toning," he said. "We can add that to our list of special areas we want to focus on so they'll look better once the fat comes off."

With a smile in her voice, she said, "I guess I'm OK about exercising specific areas that really need shaping."

"I don't seem to be as deep in trance as I was before," he said. "Let me do the 'three, two, one' to help me get back into trance."

"Good idea," she said.

"Three, BLINK, BLINK, BLINK, going down, down, down.

"Two, BLINK, BLINK, down deeper and deeper.

"One, BLINK, down deeper.

"Blinking normally now."

She could hear his breathing change and said, "Back to the staircase. Take a deep breath, and as you exhale, go down a step.

"Five. Imagine and narrow your focus to your chest.

"Notice how it gently moves each time you breathe.

"Breathe.

"And as your chest moves, imagine it changing to your desired size and shape.

"Gently exercise and tone the muscles in your chest to create the physical appearance that is natural and attractive for you. See it change now."

After a brief pause, Jean asked, "What do you want your chest to look like? You don't need to respond out loud, just think about it."

John said smiling, "That was my question."

"OK smarty," she said. "Do it again. Just tense your chest muscles slightly and then let them relax. Close your eyes and imagine your chest changing to the size and shape you want."

"Breathe," she said.

"That was different," he said. "In my mind, I flexed my face, arms, and chest muscles like I was posing for a muscle man photo."

"I'm not telling what I imagined," she said.

"OK enough of that. We need to move on to our stomachs and lower backs," he said.

"Are you sure?" she asked.

John groaned and then said, "I'm sorry, I've come out of trance again and I think it's your fault. I'll repeat the 'three, two, one.'"

"Three, BLINK, BLINK, BLINK, going down, down, down.

"Two, BLINK, BLINK, down deeper and deeper.

"One, BLINK, down deeper.

"Blinking normally now."

Jean picked it up from there and said, "Back to the staircase, take a deep breath, and as you exhale, go down a step.

"Four. Imagine and focus on your stomach area, waist, and lower back.

"Imagine removing the excess fat around your stomach area, waist, and lower back and seeing the change to your desired slim and trim size and shape.

"See your waist exactly as you want it. View it from the front, from the side, from the back.

"Gently tense and relax the muscles around your stomach area, waist, and lower back muscles. Mentally exercise and tone your muscles to create the physical appearance in your waist that is natural and attractive for you. See the change now.

"Breathe."

John spoke first and said, "This is where I need the most work. What's interesting to me is that a stomach is only about the size of your fist. Everything else that we call our stomach is really just belly fat."

"I know," she said. "But this is really an area we both need to focus."

"Then let's keep going down and focus on our hips," he said.

"Take a deep breath," she said, "and as you exhale, go down a step.

"Three. Imagine and focus on your hips.

"Imagine removing the excess fat and seeing them change to your desired slim and trim size and shape.

"Gently tense and relax the muscles around your hips. Now mentally exercise and tone them to create the physical appearance that is natural and attractive for you. See the change now."

"OK," she said, "I'm doing this one again but with my eyes closed. First, I'm tensing them slightly and now letting them relax. Now I'm mentally exercising and toning them and imagining seeing and feeling them change to become slim and trim.

"Next up are our legs," she said. "Maybe it's the way fat is distributed on women, but I seem to have a larger deposit there than you do."

Smiling he said, "Yes, I believe you're right."

"Oh, shut up," she said.

"Hey, you brought it up," John teased.

"Here we go, take a deep breath, and as you exhale, go down a step," she said.

"Two. Imagine and focus on your legs.

"Imagine removing all the excess fat and seeing them change to your desired slim and trim size and shape.

"See them from the front, from the side, and from the back.

Reinforce Your New Body Image

"Gently tensing and relaxing the muscles in your legs. See and feel the muscle tone under your skin. Imagine creating the physical appearance that is natural and attractive for you. See the change now."

"That felt good," John said.

"When we were doing this earlier today," she said, "I initially had trouble with how to tense and relax my shins and calves. Then I figured out that you can point your feet up to tense your shins and point your feet down or raise your heels to tense the muscles in your calves. Or, you could just flex all your leg muscles including your knees and thighs at the same time."

"Oh, yeah," John said. "I can really feel that."

"When my thin person emerges, I'm going to have some really nice looking legs," she said.

Smiling, John said, "Time to move on."

"OK," she said.

"Take a deep breath, and as you exhale, go down a step.

"One. Imagine and focus on your ankles, feet, and toes.

"Imagine removing any excess fat and then seeing them change to your desired slim and trim size and shape.

"Look down at your ankles and feet. Imagine them as you want them to look and feel. In your mind, stretch and move your toes. Feel good.

"Tensing slightly, now relaxing, closing my eyes so I can more clearly imagine them changing to the size and shape I want."

"Holding on to the handrail, take a deep breath, exhale, and go down into the room at the bottom of the staircase.

"Notice the full-length mirrors, the open clothes closet, the tall table with the book and pen, and the large door in between.

"I really want to imagine what I look like from head to toe," she said.

"I'm staying quiet," he said. "You're on a roll."

"Hush then," she said. "I'm going to my closet and selecting this awesome dress I've always wanted to wear.

"Imagine that you're looking directly at your body in a mirror like they have at the store where you can see different reflections of yourself. View yourself from the front, the side, and the back," she said. "Let's close our eyes and really clarify that image."

Jean paused while they both closed their eyes to fully build the imagery.

"Now," she said, "move around and feel how effortless and easy your movements have become. Notice how good your posture has become.

"Imagine what it feels like to look good in your favorite clothes. Feel those clothes on your body. Smell how fresh they are. Feel yourself moving in them. Sense how comfortable they feel all over your body.

"Ask your subconscious mind to support your belief that this is the true you. Look into the mirror and make sure the reflection you see is exactly as you imagined it. What you see is what the subconscious mind understands you want."

John broke the silence when he whispered, "Jean, I just felt total acceptance of this body I want. That's was so weird. It was like something happening deep inside me that spread to my entire body."

"So it is possible that your subconscious mind is going to support you achieving your ultimate size and shape goal after all," Jean said. "I just knew it would happen for you."

"That was really different," he said.

"Ready to ask what you need to do to help make this new you a physical reality," she said.

"Yeah," he said. "I'm going back to the point where I asked if it believed to see if I get another positive indication and then I'll ask for guidance."

"Good idea," she said. "I'll do the same."

"Here we go," he said. "Three, two, one, down deeper and deeper, down deeper."

A half minute later, Jean asked, "Did it work OK this time?"

"Yeah," he said. "It was a little different this time, but I got the positive response again."

"What about the question concerning what you should do to help achieve the goal?" she asked.

"I got more weird stuff," he said. "It was very clear that I was to keep doing what you and I are doing and that I need to strengthen my belief that what we're doing is the right way to make it happen."

"That's a coincidence," Jean said. "I had a similar message that said what we're doing would help me discover deep issues that I am to resolve to move on to the next phase. Cryptic enough?"

"I think so," he said. "We've been in and out of trance enough tonight. Let's get ready to start back up the staircase. I don't think I need to use the three, two, one, deeper down. Oh, I think I just did."

"Let me read this," she said. "Here we go."

"Go to the staircase, reach out, and hold the handrail.

"And now, ready.

"Go up to step one in your slim, trim, physically fit body. It's yours now and forever.

"Go up to step two. Feel grateful that your subconscious mind understands and believes in what you want and is now taking action to bring it to physical reality.

"Go up to step three. Notice how your feet, legs, and hips look and move as you go up the stairs.

"Go up to step four. Observe your stomach, waist, lower back. Watch your muscles moving.

"Go up to step five. See your chest moving as you breathe. It's just as you want it to be.

"Go up to step six. Notice your hand on the handrail. Watch your arms move.

"Go up to step seven. See your shoulders and back, muscles toned and moving smoothly.

"Go up to step eight. Observe your jaw and neck. See how they look. They are just as you want them to be.

"Go up to step nine. Notice the smile on your slim, trim face.

"Go up to step ten. Now mentally step back into your body and feel wonderful about the experiences you're having.

"I think we're there," Jean said.

"I feel out of trance," John said. "But Dr. Bob said that we should always be sure so I'll do a short version of the wake-up steps."

"You're right," she said. "Go ahead."

John said, "One, waking up now. Two, coming up and back into the present time and place. Three, totally awake, alert, feeling good."

"That was so wonderful," she said.

"Yeah," he said. "That was incredible. You've got a great imagination."

"Once I got into it, my imagination just took off," she said. "I smelled the new clothes, felt the texture of the fabric, felt the tightness of my skin, and saw the shape of things to come. For the first time, I recognized the thin person in me under all this extra fat. I finally saw me clearly as being slim and trim with good muscle tone."

Reinforce Your New Body Image

"It was truly mind opening," he said.

"Something else happened while we were doing this," she said. "I really feel relaxed now. I guess tensing and then relaxing our muscles let me tell the difference between tension and relaxation."

"Maybe if we did this when we're ready to go to bed, we would get rid of the stress of the day and be able to fully relax so we can sleep better," he said.

"Great idea," she said. "It doesn't matter which body parts we lump together, just that we systematically 'slightly tense,' 'deeply relax,' and 'fully imagine' each group."

"That worked well for me," he said.

"And to help with the 'imagine' part," she said, "I think we should add to our collection a lot more pictures from magazines and build a collage of people with bodies like those we're making for ourselves doing the kinds of things we like to do, or would like to do when we reach our weight, size, and shape goals."

"That's a great idea," he said. "That will keep our goals front and center. Nothing like a constant reminder to keep our priorities straight and our visions of our future clear."

"I'll pick up some poster board to tape them on so we can look at them a lot," she said.

"Let's call it a night," John said. "I'm still so relaxed, I won't have any trouble sleeping the whole night through."

"Me, too," she said. "We can do this a few more times this week using the hypnosis script to make sure we have it right and then we can try it while we're in bed with our eyes closed."

"That will be interesting," he said. "But I still want to go through the process with you talking about it as we've done so that we stay coordinated and can share any discoveries."

"Yeah, I'm good with that," she said. Maybe after we've done it a few times, we can do it by ourselves and then at the end share what we've learned."

"That would cut down on the number of times we almost come out of trance and might make it flow better," he said. "Yeah, I like that idea."

John and Jean packed it in and did indeed sleep very soundly the entire night.

Chapter 6 **Undermine Your Belly Fat**

Several nights later, John and Jean once again knocked on Betty and Ed's door. Betty said she really liked having everyone over and that it was convenient for Bob since he lived in their building. After greetings and refreshments, everyone took their familiar seats.

Bob started by asking if anyone had any questions or comments from the previous meeting or the hypnosis activities they'd been doing.

John said, "I can tell you there were many times that I felt I was completely out of trance, but then when we did the three, two, one, count down, I dropped right back in."

"The first few times we did this it was hard to tell if we were in or out," Jean said. "But now we're definitely going solidly into trance and can notice the difference when we're in or out, especially when we pause to talk. But we can really tell the difference at the end when we read the script to bring us completely out of trance."

"Were there times when you were talking that you created images of what the other person was saying?" Bob asked.

"Yeah," John said. "Sometimes the questions Jean asked me, like what I wanted my face to look like, made me have to imagine what she was asking before I could answer."

"Good," Bob said. "Those types of interactions induce what are called micro-trances so even if you did come completely out of trance, they would put you momentarily right back in."

"And micro-trances are?" Ed asked.

"These are very brief trance states that take place during a moment of confusion, or intense emotion, or trying to imagine the answer to a question, or focusing on an engaging conversation or monolog, whether you're a part of it live or reading it later," Bob said. "Most often you don't even know when they happen."

"Is that like what we talked about where we would go into trance when we read a book?" Betty asked.

"Or having an engaging conversation about what we're experiencing?" John said.

"Yes to both," Bob said. "Other questions, comments?"

"When John and I started actually tensing and relaxing our muscles," Jean said, "we felt so relaxed afterward that we fell into a deep sleep."

"Yeah," John said. "It was helping us release a lot of tension but it also seemed to calm us as well, like we were also dumping a ton of stress. It felt good. Can you give us any more pointers about how to deal with stress?"

"Anybody else get stressed?" Bob asked and then quickly added, "That's a joke."

"Seriously," Ed said, "can you reach into to your bag and come up with some help in that area? I think we could all use it."

"Sure," Bob said. "When you experience stress, your body reacts by sending out chemicals to increase your appetite for sweet or salty high-calorie, low nutrient foods that are high in simple carbohydrates. These are the so-called comfort foods."

"That's me all the way," John said.

"These types of foods spike insulin, which then converts calories into fat. Cortisol is also released as a part of the adrenalin package of chemicals. It stores that fat around the mid-section of your body that we all refer to as belly fat.

"The more prolonged the stress, the greater the amount of belly fat you create. The stressors can be a series of small events or just one large event. It's one stress piled on top of another and it all adds up."

"So to stop adding belly fat," Ed said, "we'll have to reduce the amount of stress we're experiencing?"

"That would definitely help," Bob said. "Some stressful events you can't control. But you do have control over how you think and feel about them, and that's what controls how your body reacts to them."

"Is this going to be stressful to learn about?" Ed asked smiling.

"Let me break it down for you into five stages called the stress response process," Bob said.

"The first stage is the triggering event. Something happens or doesn't happen that catches your attention.

"During the second stage, you decide if it's a good or bad thing.

"In the third stage, if you decide it's a bad thing, then you automatically trigger negative emotions that drain your mental and physical energy.

"This moves you into the fourth stage where you experience lots of physical reactions, including decreasing your immune system's effectiveness, increasing blood supply to your large muscles preparing you for fight, flight, or freeze, slowing your ability to metabolize fat while at the same time increasing insulin to convert calories to fat and cortisol to put that fat on your belly."

"That fourth stage sounds like a ton of trouble," John said.

"Yes, it is," Bob said. "It's the result of missing opportunities to weaken or shut the stress response process down during the first three stages. But not to worry. There are effective coping strategies you can use with this stage."

"I'm almost afraid to ask about the fifth stage," Ed said.

"This one isn't so bad," Bob said. "This stage is called the behavioral stage because at this point you have an excess of energy you can expend for good or bad. On the plus side, it gives you the opportunity to take care of a lot of the earlier issues that could have prevented this whole stress response process from happening in the first place."

"Now what?" John asked. "How do we cope with the stress?"

"Every one of us has to continually learn new appropriate and effective ways to cope with stress," Bob said. "Let's take a look at some general coping strategies that you could apply to your specific situations."

"We're listening," Ed said.

"To keep it orderly," Bob said, "let's match each stage in the stress response process with a corresponding set of coping strategies."

"I like that idea," Betty said.

"Good," Bob said. "Sometimes these stages can happen really fast, and we don't get a chance to cope with one at a time. Other times they may take more time and you can intervene with a solid coping mechanism at each stage.

"The first stage triggers everything else that follows. This is the stage where some event happens or does not happen that catches your attention. The event could be internal or external."

"Internal?" Betty asked.

"It could be reminiscing about something that brings up stressful memories or having a physical pain that concerns you," Bob said.

"OK," Betty said. "I see what you mean."

"Now you may not know if any particular event will cause a stress reaction, but from your own history you know the types of things that get to you."

"I can make a pretty long list," Ed said.

"That's a really good idea," Bob said. "The first level of coping is to identify the things that cause you stress and get rid of them, fix or replace them, avoid them, get away from them for a while, or just accept them and use them to motivate you so you can get on with your life. You can take action as they occur or you could make a list and take care of them before they have a chance to stress you."

"I never thought about getting rid of the stuff that aggravates me," Ed said. "That just makes so much sense."

"Let me tell you what happened to me earlier today," Betty said. "I was trying to use that old worn-out can opener I've had forever and every time I do, I get so upset with it. Getting a new one is such a simple thing and just so easy it's silly."

"You really zeroed in on it," Bob said. "You're going to be amazed at how much stress you experience every day just because you didn't think about dealing with the cause."

"I guess that means that every time I sense stress I should back up and find out what the cause is and then decide what do to about it," Jean said.

"I think we should try to deal with some of the more obvious stuff before it gets to us," John said, looking at Jean. "Let's get our own list together and see what we can deal with ahead of time."

"You're right," Jean said. "There's no sense in waiting for something we know is going to happen and cause us stress when we can take care of it now."

"But sometimes none of those first-level options of getting rid of it, fixing it, or the other ideas are going to work," Ed said. "What then?"

"That moves you on to the second stage of the stress response process," Bob said. "This is where you decide if the event is good or bad or some combination of the two. So the goal of the second level of coping strategies is to change how you perceive things from negative to neutral to positive."

"How does that work?" Betty asked.

"Just by making a list of things that stress you," Bob said, "you've already entered stage two by deciding they've got your attention and are causing stress."

"So how do we start coping once we decide something is stressing us?" Ed asked.

"The very first thing to do with any item that makes it to your list is to ask yourself if it's really worth your time, energy, and effort to deal with it," Bob said. "If it's not, dismiss it and clear it from your mind. You can always add it back later if it starts irritating you again."

"I guess there are enough important things we have to deal with that we don't need to be spending time on stuff that really doesn't matter," John said.

"That's true," Bob said. "But also consider when you're setting your priorities to put at the top of the list to clean up as many of these minor irritating things as you can first. Stress is cumulative. A lot of little, easy-to-handle stressors add up. Take care of them as soon as you can, and your life will be noticeably better immediately."

"Can we put some holidays on the list?" Jean asked. "Now don't get me wrong, I love decorating my shop and getting it ready for all the different holidays, but sometimes it can be so incredibly stressful I just want to scream."

"Absolutely," Bob said. "Holidays can be stressful and so can getting a promotion at work or making a major purchase like a home or a car."

"Oh, great," Ed said. "Now we've got happy stress to deal with, too?"

"Good stress," Bob said, "helps motivate us and keeps us sharp with positive energy flowing through us. That's a good thing."

"But holidays can be so stressful, too, and not in a good way like Jean was saying," Betty said.

"I totally agree," Bob said. "Sometimes you're really up for an event and it's all good and other times, you may have other things going on that make that holiday a stressful event."

"Does this now send us to stage three?" Ed asked.

"Not yet," Bob said. "Remember at stage two you have to decide if the consequences of the event will have a good or bad effect on you or someone or something you care about. Along with that, you will also need to decide if there is enough good stuff that happens as a result of a bad event to counterbalance and neutralize it or even turn it positive."

"If we decide it's a bad thing," Ed said, "how do we then get to the good counter-balancing stuff so we don't go off to the next stages?"

"One way would be to look for the silver lining in whatever happens," Bob said.

"That's from the old saying 'every cloud has a silver lining,'" Betty said.

"Yes, it is," Bob said. "And there is always a silver lining. It may not be apparent to you at the time, but at some point, it will make itself known. You just have to believe it's there, keep looking for it, and you will eventually find it."

"In my situation," John said, "that's going to be pretty hard to do. I don't see much of a silver lining in any of the clouds over my head."

"Maybe not right now," Bob said. "But imagine moving ahead in time to a year from now when you're slim and trim, what good might come of your efforts then?"

"Everyone I know would be asking me how I did it," he said. "I guess that would be a really good feeling to be able to guide others to achieve this."

"See, right then you saw yourself in the future and it made you feel pretty good," Bob said. "This year will pass regardless of what you do. Why not make it work for you?

"When you change your thoughts about an event, you change how you feel about it, and this will change the physical reaction your body has to that event."

"I can see myself being slim and trim a year from now," Jean said. "And as you said, this year is going by and it's really up to us to use it or lose it."

"But I still don't know if I can find something positive from every bad thing that happens," Ed said.

"Maybe there is nothing good about the event or situation and there's no silver lining for you, at least not right when it occurs," Bob said. "Maybe the only silver lining is for others who benefit from those stressful events that darken your door."

"Like a parent whose child is suffering and they go on to start a campaign that saves hundreds of other children," Betty said.

"Or a neighborhood tragedy unites the families to a cause," Jean said.

"Yes," Bob said. "Sometimes the most difficult thing about finding something positive is to know that you have to look for it."

"I'm not following," Ed said.

"Let me demonstrate," Bob continued. "Take a quick look around the room and count the number of things you see that are blue or have blue in them."

Bob paused for a few seconds and then said, "Good, now close your eyes and tell me the number of things you counted that were green?" he asked.

"Whoa," John said. "I know I saw green things, but you asked that I look for the color blue."

"I did," Bob said. "When you looked for the color blue, you found it. And you did what I asked you to do with it, which was to count the blue items. You saw green things, but your memory is hazy about them because I didn't ask you to look for them or do anything with them if you did happen to see them."

"I'm not seeing the point," Ed said.

"Have you ever bought something like a car and as soon as you drove it off the lot, you started seeing the same make and model everywhere?" he asked.

"Yes," Ed replied.

"Oh, yeah," John said. "In fact, one car I bought I thought was so unique until I started driving it. Even the color was common."

Jean said, "That happens with clothes I buy. As soon as I put them on and walk through the mall, I start seeing lots of people with the same outfit or something very similar with same colors and style. It just infuriates me."

"The reason this happens," Bob said, "is because you have a set of small organs in your brainstem that forms what's called the reticular activating system. Its job is to filter out what you don't need to pay attention to so you don't get overwhelmed while at the same time, open channels to pre-alert parts of your brain that information is coming in that it needs to handle. It opens the channel for the object of your focus. For example, things with the color blue in them. It alerted the color center, the counting center, and other relevant areas. It also filtered out non-relevant information, like those things that were not the color blue."

"Well, we'd have to know what it looked like before we could find it," John said.

"To a very large extent, you only need a broad-based description or direction to look," Bob said. "Have you noticed how some people always seem to find the negative side of just about anything without even trying?"

"Oh, yeah," Ed said. "I know a lot of people at work that as soon as someone comes up with an idea, they come up with a lot of reasons why it won't work."

"So going negative without guidance is pretty common," Bob said. "What's more difficult is to find the ways to make something work. Or, in what we're talking about, find the positive or the good that can come from the event. Ask yourself, 'Who can benefit from this?' or, 'What can I get out of this?' Sometimes that may even be years later, but it is there. You just have to keep looking for it and be open to it when it comes to you."

"Find the silver lining," Betty said.

"Yes," Bob said. "If you look for the color blue, you'll find it sooner or later. If you look for the good or look for the bad, you'll find what you're looking for sooner or later. If you can learn how to look for the good as a priority, it won't take long for that habit to take over and really make a positive impact on your life."

"Even if it's the better of two bad things," Ed said.

"Good point," Bob said. "To help you put things in perspective, you could ask yourself, 'What's the worst thing that could happen?' and, 'What are the alternatives?' Good and bad are relative terms. Once you've established the worst thing, then all the alternatives make the consequences of the event look better and help you gain a more positive perspective."

"Prepare for the worst and hope for the best," Ed said. "I think that's how that saying goes."

"One quick caution," Bob said. "Do not continue to rethink a situation in negative terms because that will only serve to re-excite your stress response, insulin, cortisol and all."

"I think because I keep going over and over in my mind how bad it's gotten for me at work I've been re-exciting a lot of stress," John said.

"If you can stop ruminating over how bad something is, the stress chemicals will flush out of your body in just a few minutes with minimal damage done," Bob said. "But if you continue to re-excite the stress response time and time again, that's where you'll produce lots of belly fat."

"I understand," John said. "I'm also feeling better because with the lists Jean and I are going to make and the actions we're learning to take, I can tell that my whole approach to dealing with stress is changing."

"My rule of thumb for this stage," Bob said, "is to always go for the positive side. Get good at finding the silver lining."

"I guess if I have a choice, it makes sense to take the one that doesn't add to my belly fat," Ed said.

"We're not talking about all stressors at all times," Bob said. "There are some stressful events where you're better served by grieving the loss first and go through the entire stress response process before you start looking for the silver lining. Make that an activity for the last stage."

"That helps put the types of stressors we're talking about into perspective for me," Jean said.

"The whole purpose of our discussion here is to find those many everyday stressors that fight your weight control efforts and deal with them before they deal with you," Bob said.

"So we're really looking to reduce the number of things that could trigger the physical response that causes belly fat," Ed said.

"Think about the first two stages as your way out of most stress you experience on a day-to-day basis," Bob said. "Save up your adrenalin rush for the really important stressors where you can't see any way around or that are life changing."

"Even for my situation," John said, "I only have one that's big like that and I think because of what I'm learning here I'm going to be able to reduce how much it affects me."

"Good," Bob said. "Let's move on to the third stage of the stress-response process and that's your emotional response.

"At this point, you're dealing with a situation you decided is a bad thing, and even though you've started to lessen its total impact by knowing there is a silver lining, you're now experiencing some really negative emotions."

"How does it matter if we have a negative or positive emotional response, aside from feeling bad and the other feeling good?" Ed asked.

"Negative emotions can deplete your physical energy and make it hard to even get out of bed and they drain your mental desire to handle any stressful issues. They demotivate your efforts to cope. On the other hand, positive emotions make you feel good and increase your mental and physical energy, enabling you to cope more effectively."

"So what's the general plan here?" Ed asked.

"If you can shift from negative emotions to positive ones, then you can minimize the negative physical effects on your body," Bob said.

"I guess I could think happy thoughts or get away from it and find something that's more uplifting?" Betty asked. "But isn't that just running away from your problems?"

"It could be," Bob said. "But it could also be first aid for stress. For example, if you catch yourself experiencing an emotion you don't like, recall what you were thinking when you felt it. Thought precedes emotion. To change the emotion, change your thoughts. When your emotions change, so do your physical reactions and that's the whole purpose."

"I like using positive affirmations to inspire me," Betty said.

"That's right on target with what we're talking about," Bob said. "You can also simply take a deep breath and tell yourself that you're calm, relaxed, and in control of how you respond to this situation. Tell yourself that you can handle this."

"What if it's a bigger problem than we can personally handle?" Ed asked.

"In the normal course of everyday events, that doesn't happen very often, if at all," Bob said. "Everyone's psychological makeup has built-in protective circuitry such that your brain will only let you perceive the magnitude and complexity of a problem at the level of which you are capable of successfully handling. And it will only allow you to fully perceive the problem when you're ready to handle it."

"So if it's a really big problem beyond our individual capabilities and we're able to grasp the full impact it has, we can work with others to solve it," Ed said.

"And recognizing you need help means that perception was within your capabilities," Bob said. "Getting help when it's needed is clearly another healthy way to cope successfully at this stage of the stress response process. Call on your support network. You can talk it out, explore different perspectives, and release emotions in a safe place, so you can move into rational problem solving during the last stage."

"And if that isn't working?" Ed asked.

"Get professional help," Bob said. "If your transmission breaks and it's beyond your ability to fix it, hire a professional mechanic trained to deal with that problem. If you're suffering mentally or emotionally over a problem, see your neighborhood counselor or support organization.

"The point is that if you can perceive the problem and it's beyond your capabilities, don't flail about. Get professional help. Your ability to see you need help is part of your brain trying to tell you that it's OK to do so."

"Getting the right perspective seems to be a key strategy," John said. "If we decided something is no big deal, then it won't send us into emotional distress, but if we're there already, we can talk it out with our friends and then we might learn how to look at it from a different perspective altogether."

"That's definitely on target," Bob said.

"Here's my rule of thumb for the third stage," Bob said. "Smile when you sense any emotion, positive or negative. Make it reflexive whether you feel it or not."

"Smile?" Ed asked.

"When you smile, you're signaling to your subconscious mind that you are looking for a positive way to cope with the stressor," Bob said.

"OK, let me see if I've got this so far," Ed said. "First we should fix or get rid of things that stress us. Even the mere action of writing them down moves us to stage two where we have to decide if they're good or bad. If we decide it's bad, we should remain optimistic that good is there somewhere, and we should smile as we enter the third stage of positive and negative emotions. Doing all this will lessen the emotional and physical toll we'll have to pay when we get to the next stage."

"Yes," Bob said. "Now let's all be clear and recognize that doing this will not be 100 percent doable 100 percent of the time, but just imagine how different your lives will be if you could tackle most of the everyday stress you encounter this way?"

"I suspect we'd have a lot less fat hanging around our bellies," John said.

"So it would make sense not to waste your energy to build belly fat on the petty little things that just aren't that important," Bob said. "Save those belly fat building reactions for the really big stuff."

"But important big stuff doesn't happen very often," Ed said.

"My point exactly," Bob said. "Why get hung up on something that 10 minutes from now will be or should be forgotten. Problems will continually jump in your path and that's why you develop great problem-solving skills. Put them to work so you can focus your energy on all the positive events in your life."

"I just had about a half-dozen things fly through my mind that fit that description," Ed said. "They're going on my list of things to fix or ditch."

"So let's continue on to the fourth way to cope, which is connected to the fourth stress-response process stage of having a physical response."

"That was 20 minutes ago," Ed said. "Is that where our bodies unleash the chemicals?"

"Yes," Bob said. "This is problematic because once the stress-response process gets to this stage, you're pretty much left with strategies designed to expend physical energy to help burn off the caustic chemicals released in your body."

"That sounds like a no-win situation," Ed said. "Any chance we can have a few effective coping strategies for this stage."

"Yes, absolutely," Bob said. "You could get up, stretch, take six deep breaths, move your big muscles like your legs, arms, shoulders, or tense and release your muscles like you've been doing for one of the deepening activities. Any of these will help quickly burn off the chemicals in just a few minutes."

"So that's why John and I got such intense and immediate relief when we tensed and relaxed our muscles," Jean said.

"That's exactly what was working for you," Bob said.

"How does deep breathing help?" Ed asked.

"For starters, deep breathing does everything from releasing tension and anxiety to adding oxygen to the blood. It helps burn fat and build muscle and it increases your energy levels," Bob said.

"I think I'm getting the picture," Ed said.

"When I get upset about something," Betty said. "I take a deep breath, tell myself to relax, and say an affirmation such as 'I can do this.'"

"Good," Bob said. "That's a great strategy to reduce the effect of the chemicals pumped in during this physical reaction stage. Again, the quicker you cope, the quicker you stop the formation of belly fat."

"So that takes us into stage five, which is our behavioral response to the stress?" Ed asked.

"Yes, it is," Bob said. "We are people of action. We don't sit around and mope to cope. We get up and make lists of action items to fix the problem. If there are people involved, we meet with them to work out solutions. We try to figure out how to prevent the situation from happening again, and we adapt and change as needed."

"So actually," Jean said, "at this level of coping some of the things we're doing now, we could have done at stage one and two and shut it down before it made belly fat?"

"For the type of stress we're talking about here," Bob said, "I think that's mostly true, but certainly not always."

"Bob," Ed said, "I just figured out that the sooner we deal with the stressor in the response process the more effective it seems to be."

"That's been my experience," Bob said. "Makes sense when you think about it. If you get rid of the stressor, no more stress. If you don't see it as a bad thing, no more stress. But remember also that good events like the holidays you celebrate, getting a promotion or new job, buying something big like a home or a car, or even having a birthday party can cause enormous amounts of stress."

"Maybe so," John said. "But those are the heavy stresses I'm good for. It's that negative side that just depletes me."

"That's why it makes so much sense to identify repeat stressors and make a plan to deal with them ahead of time," John said.

"I do," Bob said. "I also recognize that we can't get rid of a lot of the common stressors we face, but what we can do is some pretty effective problem solving to minimize or eliminate the effects of the stressor, especially if they're ones that are going to be with us for the long-term."

"So for my issues at work," John said, "things in my plan could include trying to put a spin on my not traveling right now?"

"Stress causes your immune system to nose dive," Bob said. "So not getting on a crowded airplane could be a good thing health wise until you get at least your weight-related stress under control."

"That makes me happy just thinking about it that way," John said.

"What about the strategies you can use for the physical stage?" Bob asked.

"I can definitely do the deep breathing and taking a short, fast walk right past the vending machine," John said smiling.

"OK," Bob said. "What about the behavioral or last stage? How you will deal with the stressor directly?"

"I think I'm going to meet with my boss," John said. "I'll explain that we're starting to see the results of our weight-control efforts and find out if there are some alternative ways I can meet my continuing education requirements while I'm getting back in shape."

"I think you've got it," Bob said.

"Identify the stressors and make a plan to cope," Ed repeated. "I like that a lot."

"Here's my summary," Jean said. "First find, fix, or get rid of stressors, second, find the silver lining whenever you can, third, smile when you sense any emotions and talk it out with a friend, fourth, move your body and breathe, and fifth, take problem-solving action."

"Excellent summary," Bob said as everyone softly clapped in appreciation of Jean's succinct summation.

"Later you'll get the chance to experience tensing and relaxing your muscles as you go into hypnosis," Bob said. "Notice the difference each time you do this so that you can become aware of stress tension in your muscles and take action."

"Anything we can do now to release the tension?" Ed asked.

"Sure," Bob said. "Everyone do this. Take a deep breath and now release it. Take another deep breath and release it. Now slightly tense all the muscles in your whole body all at once. Scrunch up your face, tense your jaw, neck, shoulders, arms, hands, chest, back, stomach area, waist, hips, legs, and feet, and as soon as you've got them noticeably tense, go ahead and relax them all. Relax them all now.

"Double check all your muscles and then relax them even more. Relax your face even more. Relax your jaw and neck even more. Relax your shoulders, arms, hands and back, stomach area, waist, hips, legs, and feet even more now. Good, take a deep refreshing breath and as you exhale, continue to relax all the muscles in your body. Breathe deeply, and each time you exhale let all the tension flow out. Breathe in relaxing, cleansing, and clearing energy and exhale any tension and stress you might still have hanging on."

"Oh, my goodness," Betty said. "That was so wonderful. I feel so relaxed."

"Me, too," Ed said.

"I like that method," Jean said, "because it didn't take any time at all and it was so effective."

"So now you have a quick way to dump stress when you're getting a physical reaction at stage four," Bob said. "It's a fast way to shut off the flow of chemicals that create belly fat."

"When John and I first discovered how much better we felt after tensing and relaxing our muscles as part of the deepening script we were using," Jean said, "I'm not sure we had any idea how much stress tension we were carrying around.

"Seems like stress just snuck up on us. Can we do this quick tension-release method every day just to make sure we're releasing the stress?"

"Yes, of course," Bob said. "Now you know the reason why many people do stretching and light exercise at the end of the day. It helps them to burn off the effects of stress. The quick tension-release method provides similar benefits. If you don't experience any discomfort, slightly tensing and relaxing the way you just did, there is no reason why you can't do it whenever you feel like it. If you do experience discomfort, you know who you need to go see."

"I feel fine," John said. "That's going to part of my midday routine.

Heads nodded.

"But," Bob said, "if you're thinking about doing anything more strenuous than that, especially given your current physical shape, you really should stop by your doctor's office for a quick physical to get the OK and to establish a good baseline so your progress can be measured."

"Bob," John said, "I really appreciate you taking this detour from our original objectives for this meeting, but I for one find it a life saver."

Heads nodded with appreciative comments being made.

"It's still pretty early so if it's OK with everyone," Bob said, "we can keep going and roll into talking about motivation."

With everyone agreeing, Betty said, "That would be great."

"OK," Bob said. "Let's take a quick break and then get right into it."

Chapter 7 **Discover Your Motivators**

As the group reassembled and took their familiar seats, Bob asked if anyone had any more questions about the stress-response process and the different coping strategies available at each stage.

"I'm sure we'll have some," Jean said. "But for now we need to make the time to build our lists and develop the coping strategies for each level that will work for us."

"Yeah," Ed said. "I think we have a good idea about what to do next with getting our stress under control, so right now I think we're all ready to move on to working with our motivators."

"Well then," Bob said, "let's talk about what motivates you to achieve your weight, size, and shape goals."

"Having a slim and trim body motivates me," Jean said.

"I think that's true for everyone here," Bob said. "What we're after now are ways to power-up that goal. You want to make it strong enough to get you started and to carry you through any rough spots along the way."

"I think we'll need that," John said. "How do we do it?"

"You do that when you identify other benefits you'll get when you achieve your goal," Bob said. "These benefits will need to be directly linked to the goal itself to have power."

"So the goal becomes even more important to achieve because of all the other things we'll get," Betty said.

"That's it exactly," Bob said.

Bob handed each of them a copy of the list and said, "Here are some examples of common motivators for weight-control issues.

"To find the ones that will motivate you, complete the sentence, 'I am achieving my goal to be slim, trim and physically fit because I want to ___.' Now fill in the blank."

- enjoy my grandkids for many years to come
- be healthy
- make my strong physical condition my body armor
- change how people look and talk about me
- feel real comfort and affection instead the false feeling I get from junk food
- get my sex drive back
- be attractive
- be attractive to my spouse
- have positive self-esteem
- feel good about me
- wear clothes that fit and look good
- travel in comfort
- enjoy eating healthy foods that taste good
- look as good as I feel
- have that 'edge' of alertness that slim people have
- create a healthy lifestyle because I just know it will feel good

"You now have some examples to help stimulate thoughts about your own personal motives that are functioning at the subconscious level," Bob said. "We're going back into hypnosis to find any motives that might be hidden from your conscious mind."

"Could my motives be on this list?" Betty asked.

"Yes," Bob said. "Whatever comes to you while you're in trance is worth paying attention to, whether they're on the list or not.

"This time when you get to the room at the bottom of the staircase, you'll go over to the book on the tall table. You'll notice that the pages are blank and you'll use the pen to write your name in the book and the question about what motivates you."

"Ah," Betty said. "The book, I was really wondering about it. Can you tell us about the door now?"

"Not yet," Bob said. "You have another job for the book before we get to the door."

"What's the question for the book?" Jean asked.

"The long version is 'what do I want so badly that I will do whatever it takes to overcome any obstacle that comes my way?'" Bob said. "The short version is 'what do I want that being slim and trim will give me?'"

"Any particular way we should write the answer?" Ed asked.

"Yes," Bob said. "It has to be in a positive direction of getting something you want. For example, avoiding disease could be flipped to staying healthy."

"So we shouldn't write what we don't want, like to be laughed at or talked about?"

"Where you focus your energy is what you attract," Bob said.

"But I really am tired of being fat and I'm tired of the way people look at us," Jean said. "That's what started this whole thing for me."

Bob contemplated for a moment and then said, "To help you understand what goes on in your mind when you focus on what you don't want, let me ask you not to think about a pink elephant on a green football field stomping a foot so hard into the ground that you can feel it shake."

Big grins and chuckles erupted from everyone.

"Did anyone not put any energy into seeing what I asked you not to see?" Bob asked.

Heads shook no.

"You had to create that image in your mind first, didn't you?" Bob asked.

"We sure did," Betty said. "I was so close to the elephant, I felt the ground shake."

"But in so doing you wasted energy creating what you don't want," Bob said. "The Law of Attraction says like attracts like. Imagine a dozen tuning forks. Two of them are the same note. Strike one and of all the forks, only the one of the same note starts to vibrate."

"By trying not to see the pink elephant, we had to first create it in our minds?" Ed asked.

"That's where your focus went," Bob said. "Whatever you focus your attention on, is what you get. In this case the elephant. Focus your energy on what you want. Not wanting to be fat focuses and tunes your energy to your fat and that's likely to attract more to you. Focus on your thin, not your fat. Look in the mirror and see the slim, trim you."

"Easy for you to say," John said.

Smiling Bob said, "John, let's try a little experiment to help with this."

"I'm game," he said.

"Notice the skin on your arms. Maybe blow a little air on your arm to feel the sensation."

"OK."

"Now feel the inside of your arm."

"What? How?"

"Just take a deep breath and relax your arms and notice what it feels like on the inside. It might help to tense your arm muscles to feel them and then just let them relax and notice what that feels like."

"Do this with your feet. Feel the outside touching your shoe. Now focus on what your feet feel like on the inside."

Discover Your Motivators

"One more, notice what your stomach and waist feels like on the outside. Feel the fabric of your shirt. Now, in a moment I'm going to ask you to tense the muscles around your stomach and hold them slightly tense so that you can notice what it's like on the inside without all the fat surrounding it. You can close your eyes to help concentrate on those sensations. Take a moment to make sure you can feel just the muscle and sense that nothing but skin covers it. Ready?"

John nodded his head as did Jean, Ed, and Betty as they seemed to have followed along as well.

"Go ahead then, tense the muscles in your stomach area, pull them in and just imagine that those muscles are now the boundary of your stomach area with nothing but skin pulled over them. Imagine that the fat is completely gone. Take a moment to fully appreciate that sensation. Now reach down and hold your stomach and notice the difference in the two sensations."

Bob paused. Slowly, faces relaxed and their eyes opened.

"That was easy to do with my arms and feet," John said. "It took a little doing to get the sensation in my stomach and waist that the fat was gone. But what clinched it for me was when I reached down and felt my stomach and it was big. It seemed strange."

"It startled me," Jean said. "It was like what I was touching wasn't really me."

"Me, too," Ed and Betty said.

Jean said, "This reminds me of what John and I did before when we tensed and relaxed our muscles to shape the different parts of our body. We did this to get a real clear image of what we want our bodies to look like. Is this the same thing?"

"It is," Bob said, "but from the perspective of noticing outside physical sensations and then going inside to notice the physical sensations of your thin body and then going back outside to feel the difference. It's especially impactful for your stomach and hips because they're easy to reach."

"It's like there are two people in my body," Jean said, "one fat and one thin."

"How do we get the thin one out," John asked.

"Let me do a takeoff on the story about the little boy, who with his grandfather's help, was able to understand how to win the fight between being good and being bad," Bob said. "So for my version, suppose the little boy misbehaved. He knew he made the wrong choice and it concerned him.

"He went to his grandfather and told him what happened and that he felt that inside him there was a struggle between a person who is good and one who is bad. He asked his grandfather which one would win and his grandfather replied, the one you feed."

"Let me make sure I get the story applied to what we're doing," Jean said. "There are two people inside us, a fat one and a thin one. In fact, we just experienced a little of that. The one that will win and emerge will be the one we choose to feed. So each time we look at eating, we have to ask ourselves, which one will we feed?"

"It's pretty obvious which one we've been feeding," John said laughing.

"Focus on your thin," Bob said.

"Light bulb just came on," John said.

After a number of comments, Bob said, "Since everyone has now experienced the outside-inside process, I'll use it during the deepening for this next journey into trance. This will help you find and associate a sense of physical reality with the thin person inside you."

"So we're to focus on what we want," Jean said. "And somewhere in our subconscious, we have motives that we

Discover Your Motivators

might not be consciously aware of that could be strong enough to permanently turn the table in our favor."

"Yes," Bob said. "It may be that you're aware of them, but they just don't register with you as being all that important until you discover their power in hypnosis."

"And we can discover this by going into trance and just asking the question?" Ed said.

"Most likely you will," Bob said. "But recognize that they may come to you after you come out of trance. Be patient and when the time is right, they will make themselves known."

"OK," Jean said. "I think we're all ready to go into hypnosis and find any hidden motivators."

"Yeah," Betty said. "I'm getting so excited about doing this I'm not sure I can calm myself enough to go into hypnosis."

"Take a deep breath," Ed said.

Betty did and smiled and said, "OK, I think I can do this now."

Bob said. "I'd like to continue to use the 'BLINK' induction method we used before. It helps with the anticipation of going into trance and that speeds up and deepens it from the start."

"Will we use the same staircase?" John asked.

"Yes, we'll use the staircase, and of course you can change it up if you want," Bob said. "After all, it is your staircase."

Smiles.

"But this time, I'll guide you through the outside - inside experience as you read along with me."

"I am really looking forward to experiencing this one," John said.

"I'm glad," Bob said. "Is everyone ready to go into hypnosis?"

Heads nodded.

"And if it meets with your approval, will you do what I ask you to do?"

Heads nodded again.

"Always know that should something require your attention while you're in hypnosis, you'll be able to come up and out immediately fully alert and ready to deal with it.

"Let's start by releasing some of the muscle tension and mental distractions by taking a deep breath and as you exhale, feel the tension flow out of your body.

"Again, take a deep refreshing and cleansing breath and exhale. Continue to breathe deeply and comfortably for a little while longer. Focus on your breathing.

"Should you become aware of any sounds or other distractions, simply notice them, let them increase your focus and concentration on this process, and then let them fade away into the background.

"When you read the word 'Breathe' on your hypnosis script, take a deep breath, exhale, and continue reading.

"Take your time with this.

"Whenever you read the word 'BLINK' on your hypnosis script, please blink your eyes and then continue reading.

"Here we go. Want it to happen, expect it to happen, allow it to happen.

"Breathe.

"Five, BLINK.

"Feeling good, focused, anticipating going into trance.

"BLINK.

"No pressure, no rush, slow down.

"BLINK.

"Breathe deeply and exhale. Focus on your breathing.

"Four, BLINK.

"Slowing down.

"BLINK.

"Open to the experience.

"BLINK.

"Going down, deeper down.

"Three, BLINK.

"BLINK.

"Focus on your breathing while you read.

"BLINK.

"Breathe deeply and exhale. In, out, in, out.

"Going slower now.

"Two, BLINK.

"Wonderful feeling going deeper and deeper into trance.

"BLINK.

"Narrow your focus to what you're reading.

"BLINK.

"Breathe deeply and exhale.

"Slower and deeper down.

"One, BLINK.

"Drifting down, feeling good.

"BLINK.

"Focus on the words you're reading, and let the background fade away.

"BLINK.

"Going deeper, deeper down.

"You can blink normally and automatically now.

"Breathe deeply and exhale.

"Whenever you're in trance at any level, you will always be able to read my words to continue through the session and reawaken out of trance when it's time to do so.

"Let's now journey down deeper by taking the staircase you've used before for this purpose. You can step down or you can gently float down the stairs.

"This time you'll get the opportunity to experience the thin you on the inside. Each time you go down a step, you'll go deeper than you were before.

"As we focus on each area of your body, you'll be asked to slightly tense and relax the associated muscles or if you have any discomfort doing that, simply imagine tensing and relaxing your muscles.

"Good, now take the handrail and sense its texture and temperature in your hand. Let's begin now to count down into a deeper level of trance.

"Ten. Take a deep breath, and as you exhale go down to step nine. Notice the outer sensation you feel on your face. Now slightly tense and relax the muscles in your face so you can physically sense them and now become aware of the slim, trim, physically fit person you are on the inside and feel yourself going down deeper into trance.

"Go down to step eight. Notice the outer sensations you feel in your jaw and neck. Now slightly tense and relax these muscles and skin so you can physically sense them and now become aware of the slim, trim, physically fit person you are on the inside.

"Go down to step seven. Notice the outer sensations you feel in your shoulders and back. Now slightly tense and relax these muscles so you can physically sense them and now become aware of the slim, trim, physically fit person you are on the inside as you go deeper and deeper down.

"Go down to step six. Notice the outer sensations you feel in your arms, elbows, forearms, hands, and fingers. Now slightly tense and relax these muscles so you can physically sense them and now become aware of the slim, trim, physically fit person you are on the inside.

"Deeper down … breathe.

Discover Your Motivators

"Go down to step five. Notice the outer sensations you feel in your chest. Now slightly tense and relax the muscles and skin on your chest so you can physically become aware of the sensation of having it just as you want it to be.

"Go down to step four. Notice the outer sensations you feel in your stomach area, waist, and lower back. Now slightly tense and relax these muscles so you can physically sense them and now become aware of the slim, trim, physically fit person you are on the inside. Notice how slender you've become.

"Go down to step three. Notice the outer sensations you feel in your hips. Now slightly tense and relax your hip muscles so you can physically sense them, and now become aware of the slim, trim, physically fit person you are on the inside.

"Breathe ... Good ... You're doing fine ...

"Go down to step two. Notice the outer sensations you feel in your legs. Now slightly tense and relax the muscles in your legs so you can physically sense them and now become aware of the slim, trim, physically fit person you are on the inside.

"Go down to step one. Notice the outer sensations you feel in your ankles, feet, and toes. Now slightly tense and relax these muscles so you can physically sense them and now become aware of the slim, trim, physically fit person you are on the inside.

"Go down into the room now and move to the full-length mirrors. Imagine your entire sculpted body just as you've now experienced it physically on the inside.

"Give your subconscious mind the clear image it needs to help you get exactly what you want.

"The reflection you see is the body your subconscious mind is now guiding you to make in your physical reality.

"Make any adjustments needed until you see an accurate reflection of your slim, trim trance-formed body. Take a moment to do that now."

Bob paused a minute to give time for any needed adjustments to be made.

"Now turn and notice the other side of the room. Go to the tall table with the book and pen on it. Open the book. The book has blank pages. Take the pen and write your name on the first page, and then below that, write your question, Why do I want to be slim, trim, and physically fit?"

"If you want, you can briefly close your eyes to discover your answers and then make notes in the book about them."

At this point, Bob paused and remained silent for a minute or so and then began the process to bring them out of trance.

"Good, you're doing fine. Breathe.

"Close the book and leave it on the table. You'll be using it again. You'll be able to remember what you wrote in the book after you come out of trance.

"It's time now to go to the staircase, reach out, and hold the handrail.

"Notice how comfortably deep in trance you've become. Each time you read yourself into hypnosis, you will find it easier and easier to go into a deeper level of trance so that you quickly achieve the level that is right for you to communicate effectively with your subconscious mind.

"Whenever you're in trance at any level, you will always be able to read my words to continue through the session and reawaken out of trance when it's time to do so.

"And now, ready.

"Go up to step one in your slim, trim, physically fit body. It's yours now and forever.

"Go up to step two. Feel grateful that your subconscious mind understands and believes in what you want and is taking action to bring it to physical reality.

"Go up to step three. Notice how your feet, legs, and hips look and move as you go up the stairs.

"Go up to step four. Observe your stomach, waist, lower back. Watch your muscles moving.

"Go up to step five. See your chest moving as you breathe. It's just as you want it to be.

"Go up to step six. Notice your hand on the handrail. Watch your arms move.

"Go up to step seven. See your shoulders and back, muscles toned and moving smoothly.

"Go up to step eight. Observe your jaw and neck. See how they look. They are just as you want them to be.

"Go up to step nine. Notice the smile on your slim, trim face.

"Go up to step ten. Now mentally step back into your body and feel wonderful about the experiences you're having.

"Good, you're doing fine. Breathe.

"In a moment, I will count you up and out of trance.

"If you want to intentionally go back to this level of trance in the future, you must agree to bring yourself out of trance when asked to do so.

"Let's start to count up so that you can easily bring yourself up and back into the present time and place.

"One. Coming up now, take a deep breath and come up now.

"Two. Begin to move your body where you are, stretch, and come up even more now.

"Three. Wide awake and back in the present, feeling refreshed, alert, and fully awake.

"Just stay where you are for a moment while you increase your alertness. Stretch a little and adjust your posture to help become fully alert."

Bob paused for a moment and then asked, "Anyone want to go first? What did your book look like?"

Betty said, "My book was shiny and had a latch like a diary."

"My book," Ed said, "looked like a ledger but instead of columns, it just had lines."

John offered that his book was like a small binder where he could add pages.

Jean said, "The book I found had a fancy covering of light-colored cloth and leather trim. My pen was interesting, too. It was an old-style fountain pen, and with it, I could write in a beautiful script like I used to do so many years ago when we wrote actual letters to people."

"Show off," John said smiling.

"The reason I asked you to describe your book is to make it more real at the conscious level so that you can better remember what you wrote and so that you'll be able to easily locate it when you use it again," Bob said.

"I think we have a book like the one I described somewhere in my boutique, and I know I've got a few of those pens there," Jean said. "I somehow feel pulled to begin a journal about what I'm learning. I think I'll get those for myself."

"Jean, as long as you're on a roll here," Bob said, "what did you discover when you asked the question? What did you get from your subconscious mind?"

"Several things flew through my mind but settled on what I really want is to be more flexible physically and be able to move my body with ease," she said. "I love the style of clothes

I wear, and they are much cuter several sizes smaller. When I get to my goal, I'm going to make those clothes look great."

"Sounds like you hit the jackpot," John said.

Jean said softly with a little worry in her voice, "There was another one that hit me hard emotionally. But I'd rather just keep it to myself until I understand it better."

"That'll be fine," Bob said. "Sometimes it takes a while to sort these things out. Especially when it carries an emotional charge."

Betty spoke next "There are two on the list you showed us that just came back to me. The one about enjoying eating healthy foods that taste good and the one about creating a healthy lifestyle really jumped out."

Ed laughed and said, "That's just like you, Betty. I can see it now when we're over at your uncle's house everyone saying, 'Look at her. How can she be so thin when she cooks such good food all the time?'"

"That's it," Betty said. "That image will keep me on track forever."

"I'm not getting any younger," Ed said. "At work, these young engineers are picking up some of the plum design and install jobs with the newer electrical systems because they're a lot more physically fit than I am. More than anything, an image came to me where I saw myself with strength and agility climbing around with the best and youngest of them."

"Good," said Bob. "For now, keep moving that around in your mind in different settings."

Bob looked at John and said, "John?"

"Our company gives presentations to our investors and customers, which I used to do all the time when I was in better shape," John said. "I too had a strong visual image. I saw myself slim and trim, casually discussing our work with a group of investors in a rather formal setting. Seeing that is just so motivating to me."

"Ed, could you do us a favor and grab some paper and pencils or pens so that everyone can jot down the motivators they've discovered so far?" Bob asked. "We'll be doing more with them in a moment, so it would be good have them handy."

Before Ed could respond, Betty was out of her chair headed for the kitchen and said, "Oh, I've got these really neat little spiral notebooks I use all the time when I'm cooking. I get them by the dozen so I have a bunch of them we can use."

Chapter 8 Supercharge Your Goals

"You've each found motivators that drive you to achieve your goals," Bob said. "The next step is to add power to them so they have sufficient strength, individually or collectively, to overcome any obstacle or setback that might put your goal at risk."

"I'm there now," John said. "I know that if I don't get back in shape, it could be catastrophic for me both health and job wise."

"That certainly sounds like a strong motivator," Bob said. "The real test, however, is if it can build an urge or create a desire in you that's powerful enough to break the inertia to get started on this journey and strong enough to keep you from backsliding."

"That's a good question," John said. "I think it would be."

"Was it the last time you tried to control your weight?" Bob asked.

"We all know the answer to that," John said.

"Even if it was," Bob said, "how we usually get blindsided is not by the big obvious things but by the little eating indiscretions we can justify making. Those are the ones that really add up and slow or stop your progress."

"What do you mean?" John asked.

"I know you and Jean have tried a number of diets that didn't work for you in the long run," Bob said. "Were you able to come up with reasons to justify eating foods you knew were not the right ones according to your eating plan?"

"Sometimes it was easy and sometimes it was more difficult," John said. "But yeah, I guess I have some pretty strong powers of rationalization."

"Well, in fact, we all do," Bob said. "They're based on a psychological process first understood by social psychologist Leon Festinger, which he called cognitive dissonance."

"What?" John asked.

"It means that when we do something we know we shouldn't have, it creates an internal conflict that generates anxiety that causes us to automatically do something consciously and subconsciously to try to justify that behavior," Bob said. "When we do justify it, we no longer feel the conflict with what we did, and the tension, anxiety, and psychological pain are released."

"My excuses are caused by this internal conflict?" he asked.

"All the time," Bob said.

"A lot of times," Betty said, "I'll justify the extra helping because it's a holiday, or it's a two-for-one offer, or I feel sad, or … Oh my, I do have lots of excuses."

"Are you saying this internal conflict is an automatic way for us to justify and even be OK with how we eat in the future, even if it's something that we really don't want to do?" Jean asked.

"Yes," Bob said.

"We're setting ourselves up," Jean said.

"If you don't recognize what's going on," Bob said, "then, yes, you are."

"Harsh," Ed said. "You're still talking so I'm hoping you've got a way for us to deal with this so we don't continue to sabotage our own efforts."

"I do," Bob said. "You're going to learn to counter that with another very powerful psychological technique."

"Please keep going," Jean said. "I'm just amazed at what we've learned so far."

"John," Bob said, "would you help me demonstrate with your motivator?"

"Yes, of course," John said.

"Good, then let me ask you directly, "why do you want to be slim and trim?" Bob asked with a little force in his voice.

"You're joking," John said. "Getting to a healthy size and weight for me is staying alive physically and work wise. Sorry I got defensive."

"John," Bob said. "I asked that question in a certain way to demonstrate how a challenge can elicit a defensive response. That combination of stating your reasoning while I elicited and connected it to the power of the defense emotions strengthens that particular underlying motivator belief for you."

"From the way, I responded," John said, "I'm much more sensitive to my job issues than I thought."

"Did you feel defensive?"

"You could tell by the way I responded that I did."

"I took your belief that you wanted to get slim and trim and challenged your reasons by asking you the one-word question, why, and you got defensive. When you did, you added the defense emotions to the belief behind the motivator."

"Yeah, I did."

"Does that belief feel stronger now?"

Thinking about it for a moment, John said, "Yeah, it does."

"Let's start by understanding that a motivator or a motive is based on a belief of why you want it, whether you know what that is or not."

"I might not be aware of why something motivates me?" Ed asked. "I just have this urge to do something?"

"That's right," Bob said. "Until you explore the underlying beliefs that create your rationale for why you want something, you may not know whether it has enough power to see you through to get your goal."

"Tell us the story," Ed said smiling.

"Let's start with the basic understanding that a belief is something you hold to be true until information you receive causes you to change that belief. Beliefs are easy to change by providing new credible information. Like getting directions to go someplace and getting 'go right' or 'go left' mixed up."

"I understand," John said. "If I believe I'm supposed to turn right and there is only a left-hand turn, I change my belief to what is reality staring me in the face."

"Yes," Bob said. "But what happens if someone challenges your sense of direction when there is no credible information to the contrary?"

"I guess I'd have to stick with what I believe until I'm proven wrong, or maybe think something else is wrong," John said.

"So when you challenge a person's belief, they would normally feel called upon to defend it," Bob said. "But putting a person on the defensive also evokes emotions, which are then connected to the belief."

"Just like you did when you challenged me?" John asked.

"Exactly like that," Bob said. "But there's more. When you attach an emotion to a belief, it's no longer just a belief, it's now a conviction. Challenge it again and it's on its way to becoming an attitude. An attitude is a belief that has an emotion attached to it, and that makes it resistant to change."

"I'm not sure I'm following you," John said.

"The defense emotions are evoked when a person's belief or behavior is challenged," Bob said.

"I got that," John said.

"When you successfully defend a belief or behavior while feeling the emotions, the two connect to each other and create an attitude," Bob said. "If it hadn't been challenged or argued about then when credible evidence countering the belief is presented, the belief could have been changed just like we talked about getting the directions mixed up."

"OK," John said. "I'm with you so far."

"The most important thing to know is that once the defense emotions are attached to the belief, the belief becomes an attitude and attitudes are resistant to change," Bob said. "The more the underlying belief is challenged and successfully defended with emotional energy, the stronger the attitude becomes and the more it works automatically to guide and direct your choices."

"How do we use these challenges to help us?" John asked.

"Let's use a couple of examples to show how this works," Bob said. "Have you ever asked yourself a question like, why can't I lose weight? Or, why did I eat that?"

Jean jumped in and said, "We ask ourselves those questions a lot."

"Now I get it," John said. "By asking questions that way we have to come up with some justification for not losing weight or eating whatever, just like in that internal conflict thing we just talked about."

"Ah, the powers of rationalization," Ed said.

"Now you're on it," Bob said. "Let's rephrase the question to use the power of rationalization to help us accomplish our goals. So the better question would be to spin it and ask, why do I want to reduce my weight? Or, why should I skip the cheesecake?"

"Like you asked me why I wanted to reduce my weight and then I became defensive," John said."

"It's the why question posed as a challenge that does it every time," Bob said. "There are a lot of different ways you can ask the why question and get the same result."

"So by spinning it, you got me to defend and justify the beliefs and behaviors that will move me toward achieving my goal," John said.

"Yes," Bob said. "And when you defended it, you used words that created the types of imagery that the subconscious mind can understand."

"We should keep challenging until we get something we can see ourselves doing," John confirmed.

"By getting to that level of clarity you are doing some mental rehearsal," Bob said. "When a similar situation comes up in the future, you'll have already practiced your response."

"That'll help," Betty said.

"Let's carry this to different examples to help clarify what's going on," Bob said. "When do you ask your colleagues, people who work for you, your spouse, or your kids the why question - when they did something right or when they did something wrong?"

"I've got that one," Ed said. "When they did something wrong."

"What are you getting them to defend? Good behavior or bad behavior?"

"Bad behavior," Ed said.

"And when they defend themselves with some emotional energy behind it, what are you creating, good attitudes or bad attitudes?"

"Oh," Ed said.

Sitting in stunned silence, Betty, Ed, John, and Jean went into deep thought about the many times they had unknowingly created bad attitudes about themselves and others.

"Belief plus emotion equals attitude," Bob said. "Once the attitude is in place, it's extremely hard to change because attitudes are resistant to change even in spite of volumes of credible information contrary to the belief. And remember, the more the belief is challenged the stronger and more automatic the attitude becomes."

"Uh oh," Betty said. "I just asked someone I work with this morning why they were always late. And, wow, did they have the most compelling reasons I've ever heard. That probably means they've been asked that a lot."

"Probably so," Bob said.

"Now for a bit more tech talk," Bob said. "The technique I've been demonstrating is called attitude inoculation. It was discovered in the early '60's by social psychologist William McGuire. It basically says that you can take a belief and make it an attitude by challenging it and allowing the defense to be successful. You can then strengthen that attitude through increasingly stronger unsuccessful challenges thereby making it very resistant to change.

"Our own experience shows that with repeated use or application, these attitudes can transition into values that automatically guide and motivate thoughts, feelings, and behavior."

"So asking questions like, 'Why don't you go on a diet?' 'Why do you smoke?' or 'Why are you always late?' we're going to get the opposite results of what we want?" Ed asked.

"Usually," Bob said. "And because you wouldn't ordinarily ask those questions directly if you didn't care about the person, or have some strong feelings about the behavior itself, you lend the emotional challenge to the question. And that's what turns it from an innocent inquiry to an attitude-creating encounter."

"I don't know what to say," Jean said. "I'm guilty, guilty, guilty. I challenge myself, I challenge John. I'm so sorry honey."

"Hey, don't be," John said. "I've done the same thing to you many times. But I understand how you feel because I feel guilty, too."

"And that's why I should defend not eating the cheesecake?" Ed said.

"Correct," Bob said. "The more you can repeatedly win that argument against increasingly stronger arguments for eating it, the stronger your cheesecake immune system response will be."

Jean appeared anxious and said, "I'm sorry. I'm feeling a little overwhelmed thinking about the number of times we've justified our overeating without knowing that we were making it easier to justify doing it again. And now to think about the number of times we've challenged ourselves and each other in a way that made us defend our overeating … it's just making me feel a little hysterical."

"I'm with Jean on this," John said. "If we now have those attitudes so firmly challenged and locked into place, how can we undo the damage?"

"I'm glad you asked," Bob said. "They can be changed."

"I think I need to know right now before I have a breakdown," Betty said.

"The quickest way to undo what's been done is to bring it up for discussion, support the desired beliefs or behavior, then challenge the person's reasoning for doing it correctly, and then wrap it up by supporting their reasons."

"I can bring it up, but what do you mean by 'support' it?" Betty asked.

"Just say why the desired way would be something you like," Bob said.

"I'm still not following," Betty said.

"Try this with Ed's cheesecake example," Bob said. "Betty, bring it up, support, challenge, support."

"Ed," Betty said. "I noticed you didn't eat the cheesecake I made for you. I know you you're trying to change your body size and shape. Is that why you didn't you eat it?"

"Well, Betty," Bob said, "that was really supportive and so you got the idea. You even gave him the answer that would help you understand why he turned down the cheesecake. Let's make it a little harder on him so he feels defensive. That way he can benefit."

"OK," Betty said. "Why didn't you eat the cheesecake I made for you?"

Smiling, Ed said, "I want to get to be slim and trim."

"Betty," Bob said. "Throw that back at him."

"I know that," Betty said. "But this is my best recipe. Why didn't you even taste it?"

"Ouch, I felt that," Ed said. "Now what do I say? She already knows why I didn't eat it."

"Go back to your size and shape goal and your motivation for achieving the goal to start looking for answers," Bob said.

"This is Betty's cheesecake we're talking about here," Ed said. "I would probably eat it and then use that other thing to justify my giving in."

"That means," Bob said, "that your motivation isn't strong enough by itself in its present state to reflexively and automatically prevent you from doing something you know deep down you don't want to do. That would be one of those self-justifiable eating indiscretions that will slow or stop your progress.

"If this is going to do any good at all, it must be challenged until you get down the bottom-line emotionally laden reasons so that when you get that question again, you can feel the emotion rising up against eating the cheesecake."

"Does that mean I could blow up with some sort of an emotional outburst?" Ed asked.

"Without rehearsal and understanding of your deeper motivation you could," Bob said. "That's why you'll get the chance to practice your responses to all the motivators you find."

"I'm really looking forward to that," Ed said. "If I can make that work, I can see how I would be able to knock out most of the fattening things I eat."

"Give me another example," John said.

"Sure," Bob said. "Let's do something totally unrelated to your size and shape goals."

"That'll help calm me down," Betty said.

"Suppose you had a child who was studying," Bob said. "What would happen if you walked up to him and asked, why are you studying when all your friends are outside playing? If you did, what do you think the child would be thinking and feeling?"

"If it were me, I'd be saying, I'm sorry, I must be doing something wrong, let me get outside now," John said.

"Yes, you would," Bob said. "So you might follow the support, challenge, support formula by saying something like, Hey, I see you in here studying. I can't tell you how proud your mom and I are of you for giving your homework a priority. How come you decided to do that?"

"Oh, that's good," Betty said.

"No matter what the response is, just support them again for doing what you want them to do. You might say, That is such good reasoning. We really like what you're doing."

"Ah," Jean said. "I'm thinking most kids and a lot of my staff would say, I don't know."

"How very true," Bob said. "Part of the support formula is to help them be successful to the challenge so you might say something like. When this happened to me, the reason I did this

Supercharge Your Goals

was because . . ., and then offer two or three reasons and finish with asking, 'Is that what you're thinking or feeling?'"

"I've done things before and I really didn't know why I did them," Jean said. "Somehow it just felt like it was the right thing to do at the time."

"That's a perfectly acceptable answer," Bob said.

"Can this backfire?" Betty asked.

"If you don't have a solid rapport with the person, then that potential does exist," Bob said.

"What do you mean by rapport," Betty asked.

"Rapport means to be in harmony with the other person, to be on the same wavelength. An easy way is to make sure you have something in common with the other person such as how you dress, similar interests, goals, or values you share. Bring those up as a way to orient the conversation."

"Getting back to our issues with size and shape," Jean said. "How do we use it to help us?"

"The more successful you are defending the beliefs that provide the logic or reasoning for your motivators, the stronger they become," Bob said. "You're adding emotional power and that converts a changeable support belief to a change-resistant attitude. And after you've used it successfully a few times, it will further change into a value that now will automatically guide your thoughts, feelings, and behaviors."

"One of my motivators is to be more physically flexible," Jean said. "How do I strengthen it?"

"John," Bob said, "support it and then gently challenge it."

"Jean," John said, "that sounds like a good goal. Why do you want to be more flexible?"

"Because I can't safely move around the store, and I'm afraid I might get down and not be able to get up."

Bob said, "Good, Jean. You described your defense in terms we could see and feel. But those reasons focus on what you don't want to have happen. Now defend your motivator with a more positive spin of what you want to be able to do when you become more flexible."

"You mean like, I want to be able to get to the entire inventory and move it around in the displays as I need to as safely as possible, and that takes flexibility."

"A little cumbersome but you got it," Bob said. "John, support and challenge that a little harder now."

"Why do you have to be the one jumping up and down moving your inventory? Why can't someone else do it?" John asked.

"Because it's my store, and I want it done the way I want it done, and I'm the only one who can do it that way," Jean said. "And besides that, it makes me feel good. It reflects who I am."

"OK," John said. "I picked up on the intensity there."

"Sorry," Jean said. "I guess that's just the way I feel."

"And now I think you understand the type of experience you want to get when you do this," Bob said. "Jean now has some emotional horsepower and clarification of her reasoning behind her initial motivation."

"I can't believe the way that came out," Jean said.

"The real question is do you feel more motivated to get physically flexible?" Bob asked.

"Don't you know it," Jean said.

"So now I want you to imagine seeing your flexible self-doing something in your store," Bob said. "Do it from the perspective of seeing yourself from outside your body. Just watch yourself do it."

"That's how I was doing it a while ago," Jean said.

"OK," Bob said. "Go back to observing yourself doing whatever it was and when you're finished the task, mentally step into your body and do it again."

Everyone watched as Jean's expression and body posture changed. She seemed to acquire an inner strength and calm.

"That was so different," Jean said. "It all of a sudden seemed so real."

"That's exactly what you want to have happen," Bob said. "Anytime you rehearse a behavior, especially one that's new or one that could be uncomfortable for you, do it from the perspective of watching yourself from a distance which could mean a few feet to a hundred feet. Once you're comfortable with it, mentally step back into your body and rehearse it again and again with as many of your physical senses as you can include, until you feel it lock into place."

"We wind up with a motivator that's both powered up and locked in," John said. "I get it."

"Not only that," Bob said. "You've also discovered the core rationale and emotional basis for the motivator making it virtually indestructible."

"I felt that so strongly," Jean said. "I don't even think I could argue successfully with myself over that one."

"Okay John," Bob said, "now it's time to support her again."

"Jean," John said, "now I think we both understand how important the store is to you. It's really become an expression of you. No wonder I like it so much."

"Mm," Jean said.

"And that's how it's done," Bob said. "Work with each other this evening to gently challenge the motivators you discovered and wrote in your books. Make sure you use the support, challenge, support formula to create the attitudes."

"Can we use several to increase their collective power?" John asked.

"Yes," Bob said. "Find and make them as strong as you can so that either by themselves or combined, they can overcome any obstacle, temptation, or pressure. With repeated use, they can become part of your value system where they operate automatically."

"Just like we would automatically make choices that are in line with the active healthy lifestyle we're creating," Ed said. "They would guide our decisions without us even being aware of their influence."

"That's how it works," Bob said.

"That will make it easier on us," Betty said. "We need time to practice this in trance."

"You've got a copy of the scripts to get into trance and deepen it," Bob said. "I left some blank lines for you to write in the motivators you want to power up into attitudes or test the ones you worked with here."

"I think mine are pretty strong right now without going into trance," Jean said.

"Ah, but you did go into trance," Bob said. "Remember that when you can bypass your reality checker and then imagine with many senses, emotions being number one, then you've just engaged a micro-trance."

"When everything faded out and all I could imagine was me in my store, I was in trance?" Jean asked.

"What do you think?" Bob asked.

"She was there," John said.

"I agree," Bob said. "But for right now since everyone is still pretty new at this, it would be helpful to go into a more formal trance just to be sure. Once you get familiar with the feelings of an attitude getting locked in, you'll be able to do it with greater confidence using the micro-trance."

"I'm in," Jean said. "I really want to nail this."

"The important part of all of this is to continue to repeatedly build your desire. You need these to be incredibly strong to carry you through the tough times on your lifelong journey to get and keep your true body. These motivators need to become part of your lifestyle. You can do that by challenging and then waiting a day and challenging it again. Begin to use full body imagery where you can visualize yourself in full possession of the motivator, enjoying it, and owning it. Do this with as many of your physical senses you can muster."

"We've got to fight for it to become a part of who we are so it will fight for us to make sure we stay who we want to be," Ed said. "I got that."

"In the end," John said, "it sounds like it will come down to whether or not we want it badly enough."

"Yeah," Jean said, "and we've got the tools right now to make sure we want it badly enough."

"Ed, Betty," Bob said. "Any questions before we break for the evening?"

"I need to let this settle before we jump back in," Betty said. "Can we just hold off until the day after tomorrow so we can have a chance to make our stress lists and work with our motivators?"

"Take all the time you need to get it right," Bob said. "There is no need to push on and miss opportunities to make what you're learning to do really effective."

"Thank you," Betty said as she looked to the group for approval which she enthusiastically received. "I'll keep in touch with everyone and then coordinate our schedules with yours when we've done the work on this we need to do and are ready to learn even more."

Chapter 9 **Create New Attitudes**

Later that night, Ed and Betty made their lists of personal motivators they had discovered from the list Dr. Bob gave them, the hypnosis session, and from what they felt would help them stay on track.

At the top of Betty's list were enjoying eating healthy foods that taste good and creating a healthy lifestyle.

Ed's list included getting better assignments, but to do that, he would need better strength and agility to climb around on the job site.

Ed said, "Betty, let's start with you wanting to enjoy eating foods that taste good."

"That's something that my family always did," she said.

"Why do you want that, too?" Ed asked.

"Who doesn't?" Betty asked.

"Why is it important to you?"

Betty sat there and just looked at Ed.

"OK," Ed said. "Let's tie that into your wanting a healthy lifestyle. What does that mean to you?"

"It means eating healthy foods and doing healthy things like getting the right nutrition from what we eat."

"What else?"

"Having an active lifestyle."

"Which we can't do if we're overweight?"

"Right …"

"Let's go back to the first question about enjoying what we eat. How does that fit in?"

"I guess if we're eating healthy and are becoming more active, then we'll have to watch what we eat."

"Does that speak to how much we eat?"

"Yes, it does."

Create New Attitudes

"Can we watch our portions and still enjoy it?"

"Of course we can."

"Would we enjoy it more if we ate the right amounts?"

"Yes."

"Why?"

"Because then we would accomplish both goals at the same time."

"Why is that important?"

"Look, you know how much I like to cook, and if I can serve what we eat in the right portions, then we'd enjoy it even more."

"Why?"

"Because we'd also be accomplishing our primary goal of losing weight?"

"Losing weight?"

"Well, you know what I mean. We'd reduce the amount of fat we're storing."

"Now we're getting someplace. What happens when we eat too much of a good thing?"

"Oh, now I see what you mean. The more we eat, the less we're enjoying it."

"Bingo."

"We don't feel good about ourselves and what we eat because we eat too much, and that's stopping us from having a healthy lifestyle."

"Bingo again."

"What's with the bingo? You never play."

"Figure of speech."

"I figured that out, and I figured out how it all fits. But it still doesn't feel strong enough to overcome my tendencies to cook a lot of food."

"Then let's keep going. Why do you want a healthy lifestyle? What does that even look like?"

"Oh brother," she said. "OK. I think it's because I see all these healthy-looking people out enjoying themselves, and I want that for me and I want that for us."

"Why?"

"You're starting to get on my nerves. But I'll stick with you on this. I think our whole world revolves around food, and I want more out of life. Look where I work, a store that sells things for the kitchen no less. I'm talking about cooking utensils and gadgets all day, and it's starting to feel like life is passing us by."

"At the risk of sounding like a broken record, why do you think life is passing us by?"

"We get off work, come home, fix a big meal, and we're too full and tried to do anything else. We have no other interests."

"What else would you like to do?"

"Get a bicycle and go for a ride, go for a walk, see a play or movie, go to trendy café and have a small but special coffee while we laugh and talk about life, set goals outside of work, do things together that will keep us active and interested in life. That enough?"

"Are those things strong enough for you to push back a half a plate of food?"

Betty looked down and then said, "Do you remember when we first met and all the things we did that helped us see each other as we truly were? It's what helped us fall in love with each other."

"Yeah. We did a lot of wild and crazy things."

"Remember when there wasn't a worthwhile festival within a hundred miles that we didn't set off to enjoy?"

"We did a lot of those. We met a lot of interesting people along the way. That's how we met Jean and John. It was at one of those home shows. I think she was looking for things to sell in her shop, and you were looking for some kitchen gadgets. That was a long time ago."

"If there was any chance whatsoever that we could move forward and start doing those types of things again ..."

"We do meet people easily."

"I don't want them to see us as fat, dull people. I want them to say, Hey look at that great looking energetic couple. I'd love to meet them. I want to be popular again."

"Bingo."

"What?"

"You really are an interesting person, Betty. And you remember that I can be, too. What I just realized is that you're afraid that people won't see us as the people we really are because we're buried under layers of fat and not getting out there doing what makes us happy."

Now it was Betty's turn to say, "Bingo."

"Did we just lose interest in ourselves and other people because we got fat?"

"I think that's a big part of why we lost interest in doing the things that always brought smiles to our faces for the same reason."

"Are you sure it's not just because we got so wound up in our jobs that we didn't have time for all those other things?"

"That's probably part of it, too. But I'm thinking about all the time we sit, unable to move because we're too full. All our energy is drained away. So what's left but watching TV or doing something that doesn't require us to physically move."

"Sounds like you're getting to the heart of your motivation for getting back in top physical shape. Is it strong enough to do what you think you need to do to keep you on track?"

"I think it is. We both used to do a lot of these things before we met each other, and I feel that my wanting to be socially active again is tied into doing the things that made me a fun person to be around."

"As you were talking just now, I began to think that maybe some of the reason I'm not getting the better work assignments is because I may not be the most fun person to be around at work."

"I know exactly what you're saying," Betty said. "Even at the store where I work, I feel like I'm getting distracted and less interested in what I do. It's like when I snapped at that girl for being late. That was probably just an excuse for how I feel about myself."

"Could be," John said. "Let's change roles and you ask me the why questions."

"OK. Why do you want the better assignments at work?"

"Because they're more challenging and show off my expertise."

"Why do you want to show off your expertise?"

"I'm very good at what I do, but lately I feel I'm not getting the recognition I deserve. I think I might not be seen as valuable as I once was and that hurts."

"Hurts?"

"Yeah, my esteem is taking a bashing. It's embarrassing when the boss goes to the other guys for ideas. He used to always come to me first."

"You said earlier that maybe you weren't as much fun at work as you used to be. Do you think that has something to do with it as well?"

"Maybe, but they don't seem to be as interested in having me along for lunch and I think it's mostly because of my size."

"Why do you want your esteem to be strong at work?"

"It's so much a part of my identity of who I am. It's a part of my feelings of self-worth."

Create New Attitudes

"I know this sounds silly, but just like you did, I have to ask the questions to get to the deeper answers. So here goes, why is that important to you?"

"My whole life I've wanted to be the go-to guy when it came to the job. Now that seems to be slipping away. I've always taken great pride in my work but not so much anymore and that bothers me."

"You want that back?"

"Yes."

"Getting back in physical shape will give you the energy you need and being assured that you can climb around the job site will spark your interest again?"

"People who are interested in what they do are interesting people. Oh, ah, I think something's coming through to me."

"Again with the question, why would being an interesting person make you more fun to be around?"

"Because if I'm interested in my work, why wouldn't I also have the energy to be interested in the people and the things I used to be interested in, which is what you were talking about was motivating you."

"Is that going to be strong enough to turn down the cheesecake?"

"Oh, that's not fair. But if we work together and watch each other's backs, I think it will be more than enough."

"I'm glad to hear you say that. I really am."

"Are you ready to see if these attitudes are locked in with our subconscious minds?" Betty asked.

"Yeah," Ed said.

"Let's just read it through together and fill in the blanks when we get to that part," Betty said.

"I think I'm going to write mine on my notepad rather than on the script sheet," Ed said.

"Good idea," Betty said. "Let me get mine and do the same."

After Ed and Betty finished writing their personal motivators and challenges Ed asked, "Are you ready to go into hypnosis?"

Betty nodded and said, "Let me read this all the way through out loud and see if I can do it at the same time."

"Sure," Ed said. "I'd like that. I'll follow along."

"OK then," she said, "let's start by releasing some of the muscle tension and mental distractions by taking a deep breath and as you exhale, feel the tension flow out of your body.

"Again, take a deep refreshing and cleansing breath and exhale. Continue to breathe deeply and comfortably for a little while longer. Focus on your breathing.

"Should you become aware of any sounds or other distractions, simply notice them, let them increase your focus and concentration on this process, and then let them fade away into the background.

"When you read the word 'Breathe' on your hypnosis script, take a deep breath, exhale, and continue reading.

"Take your time with this.

"Whenever you read the word 'BLINK' on your hypnosis script, please blink your eyes and then continue reading.

"Here we go. Want it to happen, expect it to happen, allow it to happen.

"Breathe.

"Five, BLINK.

"Feeling good, focused, anticipating going into trance.

"BLINK.

"No pressure, no rush, slow down.

"BLINK.

"Breathe deeply and exhale. Focus on your breathing.

"Four, BLINK.

Create New Attitudes

"Slowing down.

"BLINK.

"Open to the experience.

"BLINK.

"Going down, deeper down.

"Three, BLINK.

"BLINK.

"Focus on your breathing while you read.

"BLINK.

"Breathe deeply and exhale. In, out, in, out.

"Going slower now.

"Two, BLINK.

"Wonderful feeling going deeper and deeper into trance.

"BLINK.

"Narrow your focus to what you're reading.

"BLINK.

"Breathe deeply and exhale.

"Slower and deeper down.

"One, BLINK.

"Drifting down, feeling good.

"BLINK.

"Focus on the words you're reading, and let the background fade away.

"BLINK.

"Going deeper, deeper down.

"You can blink normally and automatically now.

"Breathe deeply and exhale.

"Whenever you're in trance at any level, you will always be able to read my words to continue through the session and reawaken out of trance when it's time to do so.

"Let's now journey down deeper by taking the staircase you've used before for this purpose. You can step down or you can gently float down the stairs.

"This time you'll again get the opportunity to experience the thin you on the inside. Each time you step down, you'll go deeper than you were before.

"As we focus on each area of your body, you'll be asked to slightly tense and relax the associated muscles or if you have any discomfort doing that, simply imagine tensing and relaxing your muscles.

"Good, now take the handrail and sense its texture and temperature in your hand. Take a deep breath and we'll begin to count down into a deeper level of trance.

"Ten. Take a deep breath and as you exhale, go down to step nine. Notice the outer sensation you feel on your face. Now slightly tense and relax the muscles in your face so you can physically sense them and now become aware of the slim, trim, physically fit person you are on the inside and feel yourself going down deeper into trance.

"Go down to step eight. Notice the outer sensations you feel in your jaw and neck. Now slightly tense and relax these muscles and skin so you can physically sense them and now become aware of the slim, trim, physically fit person you are on the inside.

"Go down to step seven. Notice the outer sensations you feel in your shoulders and back. Now slightly tense and relax these muscles so you can physically sense them and now become aware of the slim, trim, physically fit person you are on the inside as you go deeper and deeper down.

"Go down to step six. Notice the outer sensations you feel in your arms, elbows, forearms, hands, and fingers. Now slightly tense and relax these muscles so you can physically sense them and now become aware of the slim, trim, physically fit person you are on the inside.

"Deeper down … breathe.

"Go down to step five. Notice the outer sensations you feel in your chest. Now slightly tense and relax the muscles and skin on your chest so you can physically become aware of the sensation of having it just as you want it to be.

"Go down to step four. Notice the outer sensations you feel in your stomach area, waist, and lower back. Now slightly tense and relax these muscles so you can physically sense them and now become aware of the slim, trim, physically fit person you are on the inside. Notice how slender you've become.

"Go down to step three. Notice the outer sensations you feel in your hips. Now slightly tense and relax your hip muscles so you can physically sense them and now become aware of the slim, trim, physically fit person you are on the inside.

"Breathe … Good … You're doing fine …

"Go down to step two. Notice the outer sensations you feel in your legs. Now slightly tense and relax the muscles in your legs so you can physically sense them and now become aware of the slim, trim, physically fit person you are on the inside.

"Go down to step one. Notice the outer sensations you feel in your ankles, feet, and toes. Now slightly tense and relax these muscles so you can physically sense them and now become aware of the slim, trim, physically fit person you are on the inside.

"Go down into the room now and move to the full-length mirrors. Imagine your entire sculpted body just as you've now experienced it physically on the inside.

"Give your subconscious mind the clear image it needs to help you get exactly what you want.

"The reflection you see is the body your subconscious mind is now guiding you to make in your physical reality.

"Make any adjustments needed until you see an accurate reflection of your slim, trim trance-formed body. Take a moment to do that now.

Betty paused a minute to give time for any needed adjustments to be made.

"Now move to the tall table with the book and pen. Open the book and write the motivators you want to use on a blank page. Taking one at a time, challenge it to make sure the subconscious clearly understands and agrees that it is strong enough."

Motivator: _____
Why? _____

"Check to see if the motivator is now strong enough. If not, challenge it again and again until you feel its power.

"Now test it. In your mind, put it into action and see it work for you. Watch yourself do it from a distance and then when you get a successful outcome and you're ready, mentally step back into your body and do it again.

"Imagine and experience this with your emotions and with as many of your physical senses as you can.

"Connect this motivator to your ultimate goal of getting and keeping your slim, trim, physically fit body.

"Notice when it locks in.

"Good. Move on now to your next motivator.

Motivator: _____
Why? _____

"Check to see if the motivator is now strong enough. If not, challenge it again and again until you feel its power.

Create New Attitudes

"Now test it. In your mind, put it into action and see it work for you. Watch yourself do it from a distance and then when you get a successful outcome and you're ready, mentally step back into your body and do it again.

"Imagine and experience this with your emotions and with as many of your physical senses as you can.

"Connect this motivator to your ultimate goal of getting and keeping your slim, trim, physically fit body.

"Notice when it locks in.

"Good. Move on now to your next motivator.

Motivator: _____
    Why? _____

"Check to see if the motivator is now strong enough. If not, challenge it again and again until you feel its power.

"Now test it. In your mind, put it into action and see it work for you. Watch yourself do it from a distance and then when you get a successful outcome and you're ready, mentally step back into your body and do it again.

"Imagine and experience this with your emotions and with as many of your physical senses as you can.

"Connect this motivator to your ultimate goal of getting and keeping your slim, trim, physically fit body.

"Notice when it locks in.

"It's time now to go to the staircase, reach out, and hold the handrail.

"Notice how comfortably deep in trance you've become. Each time you read yourself into hypnosis, you will find it easier and easier to go into a deeper level of trance so that you quickly achieve the level that is right for you to communicate effectively with your subconscious mind.

"And now, get ready to go up the stairs. Take hold of the handrail.

"Go up to step one in your slim, trim, physically fit body. It's yours now and forever.

"Go up to step two. Feel grateful that your subconscious mind understands and believes in what you want and is now taking action to bring it to physical reality.

"Go up to step three. Notice how your feet, legs, and hips look and move as you go up the stairs.

"Go up to step four. Observe your stomach, waist, lower back. Watch your muscles moving.

"Go up to step five. See your chest moving as you breathe. It's just as you want it to be.

"Go up to step six. Notice your hand on the handrail. Watch your arms move.

"Go up to step seven. See your shoulders and back, muscles toned and moving smoothly.

"Go up to step eight. Observe your jaw and neck. See how they look. They are just as you want them to be.

"Go up to step nine. Notice the smile on your slim, trim face.

"Go up to step ten. Now mentally step back into your body and feel wonderful about the experiences you're having.

"Good, you're doing fine. Breathe.

"You've done well. In a moment, I will count you up and out of trance.

"If you want to intentionally go back to this level of trance in the future, you must agree to bring yourself out of trance when asked to do so.

"Let's start to count up so that you can easily bring yourself up and back into the present time and place.

"One. Coming up now, take a deep breath and come up now.

Create New Attitudes

"Two. Begin to move your body where you are, stretch, and come up even more now.

"Three. Wide awake and back in the present, feeling refreshed, alert, and fully awake.

"Just stay where you are for a moment while you increase your alertness. Stretch a little and adjust your posture to help become fully alert."

"I just can't get over the feeling I get when something locks in place," Betty said. I'm so motivated."

"I am, too," Ed said. "But you know, I had to challenge myself several times over a couple of the motivators before I got down to my true motives. When I got there, I could sense each time they locked in as an attitude."

"Something came to me loud and clear while I was doing this," Betty said.

"What's that?" he asked.

"I realized that it's really up to me," she said. "It's my responsibility to make my body the way my subconscious now believes it is."

"I'm not following," he said. "I thought that was the way we all thought about it."

Then she paused and said, "I'm feeling such a strong motivation to get myself back in shape. I have to stay on track. I have to make it.

"Even if I don't?"

"My feeling is that even though we will support each other every step of the way, it all comes down to each of us doing our own part," she said. "If one of us slips, the other cannot fall. We have to be stronger than that. What I'm trying to say is that for me to be that way for you, I have to be that way for myself."

"You are so right," he said. "In making it to the finish line with this we have to rely on ourselves to do our own part so that we can be reliable to each other. Just like a relay race. That's really a very good way to look at it."

"Ed."

"What?"

"I love you."

"I love you, too."

"Tomorrow," she said, "let's make some lists of the types of things we enjoyed doing in the past that we might enjoy doing now and anything else that comes to our minds that might be fun."

"How will we make ourselves actually pull off doing some of the things we come up with?" he asked.

"We'll challenge each other with the why question. If there's motivation to be had, that will find it and strengthen it to the level we need to get out and do it."

"Don't forget we need to work on our list of things that stress us and then develop our coping strategies," Ed said.

"Oh, you're right," Betty said. "I'm sure Dr. Bob will want a progress report on both. I know one stressor that will no longer cause me any grief."

"I can see it now," Ed said. "A new can opener from the store where you work will soon find its way to your kitchen."

"You know me so well," she said.

"Yeah I do, but now I'm done. Let's call it a day."

Chapter 10 Uncover Your Blocker Beliefs

There seemed to be a sense of excitement with the group as they settled into their familiar seats. Betty and Ed were eager to talk with Dr. Bob about their experiences with their stress control project and with their experiences strengthening their motivators. Jean and John were very interested in learning about the beliefs they held that could be stopping them from achieving their weight, size, and shape goals.

"OK, everybody," Bob said. "Let's get started. Who wants to lead off the discussion about stress?"

"Oh, I'm so ready," Betty said. "Do you remember my story about my worn out can opener?"

Smiling faces nodded.

"Can you even begin to imagine how quickly it was discarded in favor of a very simple new one I bought for almost nothing at the store where I work?" she asked.

Laughter erupted and Betty smiled and laughed along with everyone else.

Ed jumped in next, and said, "Betty and I made a list of the things that usually cause us stress and aggravation. We were surprised to see that most of them were little things, like Betty's can opener or my squeaky desk chair.

"And do you know that it didn't take us but a couple days to wipe out most of the items on that list with the fix or ditch strategy. What a great relief that alone has brought us. I am forever grateful for that single coping strategy. Oh, yeah, I did the same thing at work, what a major difference. Thank you."

"You're welcome," Bob said.

"Our experience was very similar to Betty and Ed's," Jean said. "The big difference was at my shop. Unbelievable, all the junk that accumulates, and it happens so fast. I'm thinking I'll use this or that or fix this or that. Out it all went. If I really needed it, I ordered a replacement that works. My life changed at the shop, I'm really enjoying it so much more without all that clutter."

"My experience at work was really interesting for me," John said. "Every time I noticed that I was tensing up, I would use the technique of tensing all my muscles at once and then relaxing them. It takes all of about five seconds now.

"But what was really amazing is that after I chilled out, I started looking for what stressed me in the first place. You got it, a lot of insignificant little petty stuff that made it to my stress me once, shame on you. Stress me twice, ha, that's not going to happen. OK, there were a couple that snuck up on me, but they are getting fewer and farther between."

Bob asked how the process of finding and strengthening motivators was coming along.

Betty said, "Ed and I really had both a tough time and a good time with this. We're still going through the process of finding and really determining if they can become powerful enough. We have a couple of motivators with super powers. They are almost to the point of becoming obsessions."

Ed laughed and said, "You think she's kidding? We're getting pictures and brochures of the things motivating us to achieve our goals."

"Connecting the motivator to our ultimate goal of getting and keeping the bodies we want is what's so powerful to me," Betty said.

After that, Ed and Betty took turns telling their stories about the experiences they had and when they finished, Bob asked Jean and John about their experiences.

Jean said, "John and I got almost the identical results with ours as we did the other day."

"About the only difference," John said, "was recognizing when they locked into place."

"Yeah," Jean said. "That whole process of testing the strength of the motivator was unreal at first. When I saw myself doing something from a distance and then stepped into my body and doing it again, it had such an impact on me mentally and physically."

"That was so different to see your whole demeanor change when we watched you do that last time," Betty said.

"It can be a big shift or it can be much more subtle," Bob said. "But in either case, you'll know when it happens."

"I can compare it to what happened to me when I was preparing for ski competition," John said. "I used to get this intense single-minded focus and such a feeling of concentrated intention to achieve."

"John and I only got a couple motivators to that level of intensity," Jean said.

"As more of these come up," Bob said, "and they will, add them to your list and challenge them until they reach the level of strength you need them to be for whatever behavior you're trying to motivate yourself to do."

"But we only need two or three to get us to our goal?" Betty asked.

"That's right," Bob said. "You may find that as time goes on and you experience changes in your life, some motivators may lose their effectiveness and may need to be replaced by others. But, you will always be able to find the motivation inside you to make this happen."

"I'm glad to hear that," Betty said. "Because one of my most powerful motivators is an incredible urge for personal achievement to prove it to myself that I'm capable of doing this and that has nothing to do with getting anything other than that feeling of achievement. It's so intense now."

"Internal and external motivators are both valid and usually interconnected," Bob said. "Part of the reason you challenge yourself about a motivator is to find or clarify the underlying beliefs and to make sure they're on solid, defensible ground because when you attach the emotion, that's what provides the power. And as you pointed out, sometimes that's more than enough in and of itself. Sometimes we use the external thing as a symbol of the achievement."

"Most of what Betty and I talked about was personal motivators during our challenges," Ed said.

"So we could start with an external motivator like getting new clothes, but when we challenge it, we ultimately find the internal motivators that drive it," John said.

"Now I see where the power really comes from," Jean said.

"Excellent," Bob said. "Let's take a short break to allow all that to sink in and when we get back together we can start in on the blocker beliefs that interfere with your ability achieve your goals."

After reassembling, Bob said, "Let me start with a simple definition of blocker beliefs. These are beliefs operating at the subconscious level that makes achieving your weight goals much more of a struggle than it needs to be.

"We need less effort not more," Ed said smiling.

Bob laughed and said, "Once we boil these types of beliefs down, we can put them into two big buckets, those related to getting good feelings and those related to avoiding bad feelings. They are really two sides of the same coin."

Bob then handed each a copy of example blocker beliefs and asked everyone to read them and note any that they recognized as being a part of their lives.

Blocker Belief Examples:
- I must not waste food.

Uncover Your Blocker Beliefs

- I must always clean my plate.
- Once I start, I can't stop until all the food is gone from my plate.
- I must eat three meals a day.
- I've always eaten large meals of rich foods.
- I eat to delay doing something that I don't want to do.
- Eating relieves boredom and stress.
- Eating relieves all sorts of unpleasant emotions.
- Eating is comforting.
- Fat is body armor. It protects me.
- My parents were fat, and so I'm fat, too.
- Some of the fondest memories I have about my family revolve around food.
- Eating fills the space caused by emotions that make me feel empty, like feeling lonely or sad.
- To reject an offer of food is to reject the person offering.
- I'm fat because my parents stuffed me with food as a way to show me and prove to me just how much they loved me.
- My friends and I love to eat. We socialize around eating.
- It brings me great pleasure to prepare a lot of food.
- Eating makes me feel good about myself until I eat too much.
- I somehow feel more confident after I eat.
- Food gives me great pleasure and then guilt.
- Foods with fat have more flavors and taste better.
- I eat comfort foods when I'm anxious or stressed.
- I substitute food for love and affection.
- I don't want to punish myself by imagining myself thin like I'll never be again.

- I eat when I'm overwhelmed.
- Eating with friends is fun. I don't want to stop.
- I feel hungry all the time.

"Did any of those hit home with anyone?" Bob asked.

Everyone nodded.

Jean said, "My parents always said that I would have to eat everything on my plate before I would get dessert."

"You didn't mention the starving kids in some other part of the world. Did anyone other than me hear that one?" Betty asked.

"I got that one," John said.

"Well, there are starving kids," Ed said.

Sounding frustrated Betty asked, "How does 'me' getting fat help them?"

Bob quickly interjected. "No, I didn't mention that one. In fact, even as long as this list is, there are many more of these types of blocker beliefs."

"The real question for me is how can we eat the amount of food we should be eating without getting upset or wasting so much?" Ed asked.

"Can you give us an example?" Bob asked.

"Let's say I grill some hamburgers for us and after one bite I'm done," Ed said. "I'm really having a hard time seeing me throw the rest away."

"I guess we need to be more creative," Betty said. "What if instead of full-sized burgers, you fixed the bite-size sliders?"

"That'll work great," Ed said. "Now restaurants are a different story. They seem to want to super-size everything."

"That's very true," Jean said. "But on the other hand, when Betty and I go to lunch, we've started splitting an order and just pay the split meal charge for the extra plate."

Uncover Your Blocker Beliefs

"And," Betty said, "we're seeing more and more restaurants add healthy choice or low-calorie type items to their menus."

"We can go online and look at the menus before we make reservations," John said.

Betty spoke up and said, "There's another one of those beliefs that really got me. My family really focused on having our meals together. It's meant a lot to me. Some of my fondest memories are around the evening dinner table."

"And you don't want to lose those feelings," Bob said.

Tears started forming in her eyes as she said, "No, they're way too important to me. It's what I really remember about my parents."

"It's really more about the people in your life than it is about the food, but the food triggers those fond memories," Bob said.

Betty was deep in her memories when she looked up and nodded.

"Then what we've got to do is make sure you can continue to experience those great memories and still be on your plan to achieve the body weight you want. How can that be done?"

"We don't always eat the foods I ate with my parents every day, so I guess it could even be more special if we did focus on having those meals just once or twice a month," she said.

Ed nodded and said, "I like the idea of having a special night where we honor our family traditions by making the foods that trigger those feelings. The only thing we'll have to do is to use smaller plates to control the portion sizes."

Bob looked at Betty and said, "So you don't have to give up what brings you these cherished memories, you just have to make that a special time and that's the way it should be."

"Maybe we could listen to some of their favorite music when we do this," Betty said.

"Yeah," Ed said. "I'd like that."

John looked at the list of blocker beliefs that Bob handed out and said, "Bob, I'm looking at this list and from what you said earlier, a lot of these beliefs aren't on this list. My concern is that we could have discussions like this for days to come and still not get through all of them."

Ed added, "And then we might not get to all the beliefs or at least all the right beliefs."

"That's why," Bob said, "we'll use the same process you used to find your hidden motivators to find any personal blocker beliefs. This will be another use for your books. And remember, you can do this on your own anytime you get the sense that maybe there is something else that you need to discover."

"I'm ready for a little hypnosis," John said.

"I'd like that, too," Jean said. "I somehow feel there is something else for me."

Ed and Betty nodded their heads and Ed said, "From a guy that had some doubts early on, I'm totally ready to find out what beliefs I could possibly have that are blocking my way."

"OK then," Bob said. "If everyone is ready, we'll again use the blink induction. And for the staircase deepening, I'm going to use a short version of the body sculpting deepener we used a couple times before.

"Make this one go faster when you use it so that you can check to see that the image is immediately available and clear. I'm also going to add that I want you to 'see it, feel it, own it' to the end of each statement before you go down to the next step."

"What does that do?" Ed asked.

"This will enable you to draw on your earlier inside-outside staircase experiences to ensure you get a multi-sensory impact to make it real to your subconscious minds and it will strengthen your subconscious beliefs that you own this body, it's you in every way."

"I like that," Jean said.

"Once in trance at the bottom of the staircase, I'll ask you to go to your books on the tall table and write any additional beliefs operating at the subconscious level that block your ability to control your weight and bring them to your awareness."

"I didn't bring my sheet with the 'blink' induction," Betty said.

"That's OK," Bob said. "For this, you can just imagine the sheet in front of you and that you're reading it as I say it, and each time I say the word 'BLINK' just read the word in your mind's eye and then blink.

"Are you ready to go into hypnosis?" Bob asked.

Heads nodded.

"And if it's OK with you, will you do what I ask you to do?"

Heads nodded again.

"Always know that should something require your attention while you're in hypnosis, you'll be able to come up and out immediately fully alert and ready to deal with it.

"Let's start by releasing some of the muscle tension and mental distractions by taking a deep breath, and as you exhale, feel the tension flow out of your body.

"Again, take a deep refreshing and cleansing breath and exhale. Continue to breathe deeply and comfortably for a little while longer. Focus on your breathing.

"Should you become aware of any sounds or other distractions, simply notice them, let them increase your focus and concentration on this process, and then let them fade away into the background.

"When you read the word 'Breathe' on your hypnosis script, take a deep breath, exhale, and continue reading.

"Take your time with this.

"Whenever you read the word 'BLINK' on your hypnosis script, please blink your eyes and then continue reading.

"Here we go. Want it to happen, expect it to happen, allow it to happen.

"Breathe.

"Five, BLINK.

"Feeling good, focused, anticipating going into trance.

"BLINK.

"No pressure, no rush, slow down.

"BLINK.

"Breathe deeply and exhale. Focus on your breathing.

"Four, BLINK.

"Slowing down.

"BLINK.

"Open to the experience.

"BLINK.

"Going down, deeper down.

"Three, BLINK.

"BLINK.

"Focus on your breathing while you read.

"BLINK.

"Breathe deeply and exhale. In, out, in, out.

"Going slower now.

"Two, BLINK.

"Wonderful feeling going deeper and deeper into trance.

"BLINK.

"Narrow your focus to what you're reading.

"BLINK.

"Breathe deeply and exhale.

"Slower and deeper down.

"One, BLINK.

"Drifting down, feeling good.

"BLINK.

"Focus on the words you're reading, and let the background fade away.

"BLINK.

"Going deeper, deeper down.

"You can blink normally and automatically now.

"Breathe deeply and exhale.

"Whenever you're in trance at any level, you will always be able to read my words to continue through the session and reawaken out of trance when it's time to do so.

"Now imagine that you're at the top of your 10-step staircase.

"At the bottom is the room you created where you communicate with your subconscious mind.

"Each time you move down a step, you'll feel yourself going deeper and deeper into trance. You can step down or gently float down the stairs.

"Ready? Good, now take the handrail and sense its texture and temperature in your hand.

"Ten. Take a deep breath and as you exhale go down a step.

"Nine. Form your face into the size and shape you want it to be. See it, feel it, own it.

"Eight. Form your jaw and neck into the size and shape you want them to be. See it, feel it, own it.

"Drifting deeper down … breathe.

"Seven. Form your shoulders and back into the size and shape you want them to be. See it, feel it, own it.

"Six. Form your arms, elbows, forearms, hands, and fingers into the size and shape you want them to be. See it, feel it, own it.

"Floating deeper, deeper down.

"Five. Form your chest into the size and shape you want it to be. See it, feel it, own it.

"Breathe ... Good ... You're doing fine.

"Four. Form your stomach area, waist, and lower back into the size and shape you want it to be. See it, feel it, own it.

"Going down, deeper down.

"Three. Form your hips into the size and shape you want them to be. See it, feel it, own it.

"Two. Form your legs into the size and shape you want them to be. See it, feel it, own it.

"One. Form your ankles, feet, and toes into the size and shape you want them to be. See it, feel it, own it.

"Breathe.

"Go down into the room now. Notice that each time you count yourself down, it becomes easier and easier for you to go deeper and deeper into trance and to find just the right level of depth for you.

"Move to the full-length mirrors. The reflection you see is the body your subconscious mind is now guiding you to make in your physical reality.

"Make any adjustments necessary until you see an accurate reflection of your slim, trim, physically fit, trance-formed body. Take a moment to do that now.

Bob paused for a minute and then continued.

"Now move to the tall table with your book on it. Turn to a blank page and write your question, 'What beliefs block me from achieving my weight, size, and shape goals?'

"If you want, you can briefly close your eyes to find your answers and then make notes in the book about them.

At this point, Bob paused for a minute and then began the process to reawaken them."

"Good, you're doing fine. Breathe," Bob said.

"You'll remember everything you wrote in your book so you can close it now and leave it on the table. You'll use it again.

"It's time now to go to the staircase, reach out, and hold the handrail.

"Notice how comfortably deep in trance you've become. Each time you read yourself into hypnosis, you will find it easier and easier to go into a deeper level of trance so that you quickly achieve the level that is right for you to communicate effectively with your subconscious mind.

"Whenever you're in trance at any level, you will always be able to read my words to continue through the session and reawaken out of trance when it's time to do so.

"And now, ready.

"Go up to step one in your slim, trim, physically fit body. It's yours now and forever.

"Go up to step two. Feel grateful that your subconscious mind understands and believes in what you want and is now taking action to bring it to physical reality.

"Go up to step three. Notice how your feet, legs, and hips look and move as you go up the stairs.

"Go up to step four. Observe your stomach, waist, lower back. Watch your muscles moving.

"Go up to step five. See your chest moving as you breathe. It's just as you want it to be.

"Go up to step six. Notice your hand on the handrail. Watch your arms move.

"Go up to step seven. See your shoulders and back, muscles toned and moving smoothly.

"Go up to step eight. Observe your jaw and neck. See how they look. They are just as you want them to be.

"Go up to step nine. Notice the smile on your slim, trim face.

"Go up to step ten. Now mentally step back into your body and feel wonderful about the experiences you're having.

"Good, you're doing fine. Breathe.

"You've done well. In a moment, I will count you up and out of trance.

"If you want to intentionally go back to this level of trance in the future, you must agree to bring yourself out of trance when asked to do so.

"Let's start to count up so that you can easily bring yourself up and back into the present time and place.

"One. Coming up now, take a deep breath and come up now.

"Two. Begin to move your body where you are, stretch, and come up even more now.

"Three. Wide awake and back in the present, feeling refreshed, alert, and fully awake.

"Just stay where you are for a moment while you increase your alertness. Stretch a little and adjust your posture to help become fully alert."

Everyone started to look pensive, waiting to hear what the others found out about the beliefs blocking their way.

"Jean," Bob said. "Were you able to uncover any other beliefs that might interfere with your ability to control your weight the way you want to?"

"Well," Jean said, "the answer I got was a little unnerving, and yet I understand it completely now. It was on the list that fat was body armor, but it didn't register until I wrote it in my book."

"What?" Betty asked. "Is this related to what happened to you?"

Nodding her head she said, "My answer said that when you're fat you won't get ..." Tears started welling up in her eyes. "I don't want to draw attention from the wrong type of people when we're out in public. That sometimes frightens me."

"First," Bob said, "am I right to assume that you've shared whatever happened with John, Ed, and Betty?"

Jean nodded and said, "They've heard the story many times, so it's OK to talk about it."

"John, Ed, Betty," Bob said, "are you OK with exploring this further in the context of what we're doing?"

"Oh, yes," Betty said. "If it will help Jean in any way ..."

John and Ed nodded.

"OK then," Bob said. "Jean, so you've been thinking that being heavy makes you a less attractive target?"

Jean nodded, but still appeared apprehensive. "Having an attractive body just makes me feel more vulnerable."

Bob nodded and said, "No doubt women are in a much different situation than men. Women have real physical danger to deal with, especially when it comes to predators."

At this comment, Jean shuddered and said, "I feel comfortable with the help I got back then and the precautions I'm taking now. But what surprised me was how hard that belief and those feelings hit me."

"I'm so sorry," Betty said.

With emotional rawness in her voice, Jean said emphatically, "I'm not going to let creeps like that control my life anymore. Yes, my fears are real and yes I know because of my experience I have to be extra careful, but regardless, I don't want to be fat anymore. I just don't want to be fat anymore!"

"Your need 'not to be fat' is definitely helping you push through and overcome an intense fear," Bob said. "Your anger over the control creeps have had over your ability to achieve your goals is still strong and raw."

"Yes, I'm angry," Jean said. "These fears have kept me from getting what I really want. But what's so strange is that before I wrote it in the book, I didn't realize those emotions were so strong."

"Could this be related to one of the motivators you uncovered last time?" Bob asked.

Jean said, "Of course it is. I can see that now. The motivator I saw then was being strong enough to stare fear down. That wasn't clear. But to stare *that* fear down makes it crystal clear."

"Now you can stop giving energy to their ability to block you from getting what you want," Bob said.

"Yes," Jean said, "I still have the fear of being vulnerable, but what I do know now is that I'd much rather be in good physical shape to deal with it."

"Maybe that has something to do with your aversion to exercise," John said softly.

"Hmm," Jean said. "If I'm fat and out of shape, who would want me?"

"But it doesn't work that way for me," John said. "I still love you and want you no matter what."

Jean looked adoringly at John, smiled and then said with conviction, "We will do this together, and we will be just fine."

John was out of his chair and on one knee next to her and squeezed her hand, smiled, and knew at that moment they would make this work.

Bob waited until John was back in his chair before asking Betty what she discovered.

Uncover Your Blocker Beliefs

"You know I just realized a little of the opposite of what Jean is going through," Betty said.

"Go on, Betty," Bob said.

"I was just thinking that I might feel threatened if other women looked at Ed," she said.

"What?" Ed asked. "Do you mean you've been keeping me fat so other women won't look at me?"

"No, not intentionally," Betty said defensively and then chuckled. "Well, you are good looking. Maybe it's subconsciously intentional."

"Ah ha," Ed said, "It's not my fault at all that I'm overweight and out of shape."

Betty poked him and said, "Stop that. It seems I have some fears floating just under the surface and this talk we're having is helping me clarify some things I'll need to come to grips with."

Bob asked, "Betty, did you discover anything that you were able to write in your book?"

"Not then," Betty said. "But like you pointed out, if it didn't happen in that session, it would later, and I believe it just did for me."

"That's what I thought," Bob said. "I just wanted to make sure."

"Ed," Bob asked, "how about you? Anything go into the book?"

"Yes, as a matter of fact, there was," he said. "I wrote down that part of my weight problem relates to a belief I have that since my dad was overweight, I'd be overweight. I just naturally accepted that as fact. I didn't even know I was thinking that or that it would have such a strong influence on me."

"And now you know and you'll be able to debunk what became a self-fulfilling prophecy for you," Bob said.

"I'm on it," Ed said.

Bob shifted his posture toward John and asked, "John, what about you? Anything for your book?"

"Yeah," John said. "I wrote 'comfort.'"

Bob said with some encouragement in his voice, "A little bit more would be helpful to know. John."

"I'm the poster boy for someone who loves comfort food. I've eaten myself to the size where I'm too fat to fly. That means there are some important conferences that I should attend but can't. I think that will weigh heavily, pardon the pun, on my next evaluation."

"That's a lot," Bob said.

"But," John said, "I'm really working hard with how I'm handling stress at work, and so I'm doing what I can to avoid the vending machine in the hall. But sometimes I give in and when I do, I have a tendency to get down on myself. I just get so mad sometimes."

"Stress can sneak up on us all," Bob said. "Every time you feel even remotely close to giving in, you might want to explore where that stress is coming from and then take action. Smile and say, 'when I find it, I will fix it, and it will be good for me.' It's simple but it works."

"Can I beat this?" John asked.

"There is no doubt that you will beat it," Bob said. "Sometimes awareness is half the battle. You've got that plus your strategies are working most of the time. That means some fine tuning is in order to put you over the top on success with this."

"See, John," Jean said, "I knew you were on the right track. We both just need to be more supportive and patient with each other as we learn how to use the coping strategies more effectively for the stressors we face."

Uncover Your Blocker Beliefs

"That's right," Bob said. "Sometimes it takes a little rework to get it just right and even then, it might not work all the time in every situation."

"So we can cut ourselves a little slack every once and a while," Ed said.

"I would," Bob said. "Ok, let's keep moving then toward reviewing the blocker beliefs you found and then work on developing the supportive beliefs that will counter them at the subconscious level."

"And I'll bet we'll go back into trance to communicate them," Ed said.

"That's right," Bob said. "So let's take a moment to jot down in your notebooks the additional blocker beliefs you discovered. Then we'll take some time here to find the supportive beliefs that will counter them."

"You know," Jean said. "I'm looking at what I wrote and can see that there may only be a few blocker beliefs for me. They're strong ones, but I've only found a couple. Shouldn't I have a lot more?"

"Most people will have at least one to as many as five strong ones that block them from achieving their goals," Bob said. "That also seems to be true for most goals, not just weight."

John, Ed, and Betty nodded agreement.

"Now that doesn't mean that you won't discover more," Bob said. "Sometimes your subconscious mind will hold back some things until it thinks you're ready to constructively and instructively deal with them. When they show up, just add them to your list and deal with them."

"I'm ready to start converting mine," Betty asked.

"Go ahead and tell us the ones you have now," Bob said.

Betty looked at her list and said, "The beliefs I came up with were that I have to eat everything on my plate, rich foods make me feel good, my family and food are my fondest memories, and feeling a little threatened when Ed is slim and trim."

"Let's start with eating everything on your plate," Bob said. "Who wants to take a stab at converting that one?"

"I've got one," Ed said. "That's very close to telling me not to waste food. So I'm thinking I can turn that into a supportive belief if I say, 'Take only the portions of food I need for nutrition.'"

"I like that," John said. "How about I'd rather let the food go to waste than go to my waist. Get it?"

Smiles and moans.

"The next one Betty mentioned related to fattening foods making her feel good," Bob said. "Is that because you're feeling down or sad like you mentioned earlier?"

She nodded and said, "Uh-huh."

Jean said, "Food tastes better when I'm smiling. Would it work if you were to believe that you are going to smile and look for happy thoughts until you feel positive enough to eat?"

"Then I probably wouldn't eat," Betty said. "Oh, yeah, duh."

"Moving along," Bob said. "We discussed the belief about your family associated with food earlier.

"Yes," Betty said. "I'm thinking that we'd eat our healthy meals all month and then on a special occasion we could honor them and those feelings by eating what we all ate growing up, but in the right portions."

"I like that idea," Ed said smiling.

"And that brings us to your belief about feeling insecure when Ed is slim, trim, and potentially attractive to other women," Bob said.

"I think it could also be perceived as what a lucky woman you are to have such a great-looking guy with you," Jean said. "It should make you proud that he chose you."

"You know," Betty said, "you're right, especially when it's the two of us looking good."

"Do you have what you need?" Bob asked Betty.

"Yeah," she said. "I'm proud that Ed wants to get into shape. It is as much for us as it is for him. One of the reasons we talked about getting our weight under control was so that we would have the energy and interest in going out together doing some of the fun things we used to do that brought us together in the first place."

"Circling back around to you, Jean," Bob said, "Aside from the body armor blocker belief that you've resolved, are there any others that you found?"

"Just the one about my parents making me clean my plate before they would let me have dessert," Jean said.

"So they were encouraging you to get nourishment first and that came from foods that didn't taste as good as dessert," Bob said. "Is that about how you see it?"

"Pretty much so," Jean said. "And now since I've put on so much weight, dessert is out of the question. And the really sweet ones don't taste as good as they used to."

"Taste buds change," Bob said. "Maybe its best, at least until your achieve your weight, size, and shape goals, to come up with a supportive belief for your decision not to have desserts."

"Actually I'm OK with this one," Jean said. "I now believe that I can have dessert when and where I want it. I can eat as much or as little as I want. That gives me total control over whether I choose to eat it or not."

"Ed," Bob said. "You're up."

"We've touched on the ones related to portion control," Ed said. "And I've added to that using the saying, 'Feed the thin person and let my fat storage make up the difference in what the fat person wants.'"

"That'll work," Bob said. "Just monitor what happens after a couple days. If you hit a plateau or start gaining weight, you might have cut back too far and triggered the starvation reflex."

"Good point," Ed said. "I'll eat slowly and stop when I'm near full and keep thinking about feeding just the thin person. That really talks to me."

"Eating slowly and stopping when you're near full is a great strategy," Bob said. "It could take 20 minutes before the brain recognizes that you're full and by then if you're a fast eater, you may have eaten way more than you had intended.

"One other comment here," Bob said. "I'd like you to start using your intuitive gut feelings to help you determine what food to eat and when you've had enough. The more you do this, the better calibrated it becomes and the more this gut feeling will be able to help keep you on track."

"I'm going to do that as well," Jean said. "I've always had a good intuitive feel for a lot of things and adding what, when and how much I eat seems like a natural fit."

"And if we do that," Betty said, "it won't matter where we are or what we're doing."

"I can see that's where this is heading," Ed said. "That's truly a broad-based and long-term strategy.

"It is," Bob said. "Any other blocker beliefs?"

"The one about my dad being overweight and that meant I would be overweight," Ed said. "Now I know that heredity has a minor influence and it can increase the risk that I'll be overweight, but it doesn't have to play a dominant role."

"It's not locked in," Bob said.

Uncover Your Blocker Beliefs

"This is what I'm using as my supportive belief," Ed said. "I am my own person and can control my own weight, size, and shape. My destiny belongs to me. Is that strong enough?"

"Sounds like it," Bob said.

"Some of the things that stress me no end are on that list of blocker beliefs you handed out," Betty said. "You know, some of these beliefs seem like they're from my childhood."

"Yeah, I agree," Ed said. "Does that mean childhood beliefs might be in some way responsible for our current weight predicament? But why now? They didn't always seem to have that effect on us earlier, did they?"

"I think they did," Bob said. "But they are now taking their toll because the diet and lifestyle that built your current bodies consisted of larger meals of fattening foods and a sedentary lifestyle that generates increasing amounts of fat to replace your unused muscles. Once this happens, over time your metabolism starts to slow and you gain a pound or two each year."

"That means that if we didn't stay on top of our diet and lifestyle from the beginning," Ed said, "it's pretty much in the numbers that we'd wind up overweight."

"Look around you," Bob said. "You're not alone."

"Oh yeah," John said. "I can see that."

"But also realize that these blocker beliefs don't have to come from childhood. They could come from trauma, emotional learning, significant events, gradual changes, and a lot of other things," Bob said.

"That's an understatement," Jean laughed. "We've got a lot of those things going on as well."

"Our job then is to get the subconscious mind to identify and change the beliefs that are keeping us fat to beliefs that will help make us thin," Bob said. "When you're clear with your subconscious mind that you used to believe something was

165

true, but now you know that's not right for you anymore but rather something else is true, it can then start the change process."

"It wants to know that the belief is not valid anymore but that it's going to be replaced?" Jean asked.

"Yes," Bob said. "This means that when you give it your new supportive belief, you also need to challenge the new belief so the motivation for the change becomes clear and to help get the new supportive belief locked in place."

"Help me with an example," Betty said.

"OK," Bob said. "Remember your parents wanted you to eat all the nutritious food they prepared for you. If you didn't like the vegetables, your parents might coax you by telling you that must clean your plate for whatever reason, to get dessert or because there are starving children in the world."

"That one is mine," Betty said.

"And mine," Jean said.

"So how do those ideas influence you today?" Bob asked.

"We clean our plates," Betty and Jean said in unison.

"So what would be a useful belief today that you could use to replace the one that's causing you to overeat?" Bob asked.

"Whenever I get ready to put food on my plate," Betty said, "I need to just put the right sized portions."

Supporting and then challenging Betty, Bob said, "That's a good strategy. Why is that important to you?"

"I don't want to eat more than I should," Betty responded.

"Why?" Bob asked again.

More forcefully Betty responded with, "Because I want to get my slim, trim body back that I've worked so hard to imagine and have started to achieve."

"Now you've got it," Bob said supportively.

Betty beamed.

Uncover Your Blocker Beliefs

"Jean," Bob said, "you used to believe that you had to eat everything on your plate before you could have dessert. Now when you see more food on your plate than you should eat, what belief do you need to put in place with your subconscious mind?"

"I'm grown up now and I can have whatever food I want whenever I want it and that gives me total control over whether I choose to eat it or not," she said.

"That's good control. Why is that important to you?" Bob asked.

"I want to wear skinny jeans," she said emphatically.

"Excellent," Bob said. "Now here you have two similar beliefs instilled during childhood that are no longer valid or healthy. They need to be counter-balanced with beliefs that will support their individual weight control goals.

"Betty's strategy lets her continue to clean her plate but with a lot, less damage and Jean's strategy counters the obsolete belief head on. Both can be effective and for now, that's what matters most."

"Does that mean that I'm done with that particular belief because we just worked through it?" Jean asked.

"It's possible," Bob said. "Especially if you felt really strong emotions when you answered the challenge because then you'd know that you were probably in a micro-trance. With some repetition, it could certainly reach the subconscious mind and make the changes you need."

"But not guaranteed?" Jean asked.

"If after some time has passed and you sense it's not as strong as before," Bob said, "you might want to refresh it using the attitude-inoculation technique both in and out of trance."

"It seems the objective is to make the changes at the subconscious level," Jean said.

"That's where the beliefs are operating," Bob said.

"So we should do just like we did with the motivators," Ed said. "Work them out at the conscious level, and then go into trance to make sure the beliefs are changed at the subconscious level."

"Right," Bob said. "Take your time with this. For our next session, I'll insert some of the ones we talked about in the hypnosis script for you to experience, and I'll add some others that may not be at the top of your list but might be helpful."

"That would be great," Betty said.

"Is there a format you want us to use?" Ed asked.

"Yes," Bob said. "Thanks for reminding me. I like to frame this belief-changing process with 'I used to believe,' and say the obsolete belief and then continue with, 'but that was wrong for me, I now believe,' and then state the supportive belief."

"We can write these in our notebooks?" Ed asked.

"Sure," Bob said. "And there will be blank lines in your scripts you can use to write in your personal obsolete beliefs and the new supportive beliefs there or you can certainly write them in your notebooks or in your journals. It will look like this so if you want to complete them ahead of time that would be good."

Bob gave them this format for their notes.

I used to believe _____
But that was wrong for me.
I now believe _____
Why? _____

"I'm beginning to see that there might be a benefit in the long run to have a place to keep track of everything we're doing," John said.

"My journal is really helping me keep track of all the work we're doing here," Jean said.

"When I first started doing this for myself, I used a small tablet," Bob said. "But after I really got into it, I realized I would need a more substantial way of keeping track of everything that needed to be done and so I picked up a thin bound book with blank pages from the bookstore."

"I'm getting the ledger I imagined," Ed said.

"John," Jean said. "Not to worry, I've got the binder you described at my store and will bring it home tomorrow."

And with that, everyone realized that the late hour had crept up again so they decided to call it a night. Betty volunteered to coordinate schedules for their next session. Bob said he'd have the trance script handout ready for them for their next meeting.

Chapter 11 Replace Your Blocker Beliefs

Once back in the condo, everyone was eager to take their seats and get this session going.

When the chatter died down, Bob asked, "So who's making progress on their weight, size, and shape goals?"

"We're all making progress," Jean said smiling broadly.

"What's really hitting me is how I see myself now," Betty said. "I'm noticing my shape is changing. It's subtle, but I swear I can tell the difference."

"You are changing your shape," Bob said. "Everyone here is. For one, the fat is coming off because you're paying attention to what, when, and how much you're eating. But I think what you're noticing the most is that your muscles are starting to pull your body into the shape you're imagining it to be. This is part of the image you gave your subconscious mind. So along with your growing confidence, your posture is changing for the better."

"I am noticing that, too," Ed said. "I think it could be from the extra activity I'm trying to do on the job. But it could also be a result of my military training of 'shoulders back, chest out, and stomach in' that for some reason popped into my mind."

"I didn't have military training," John said. "But even I started noticing it for both Jean and myself. I hope it's not just wishful thinking."

"It's very real," Bob said. "You're subconscious minds have already started doing what you've asked them to do. Keep focusing on your thin."

"I do that all the time," Jean said. "If I see a reflection of me in one of the mirrors in my shop, I say to myself, 'focus on your thin.' It feels empowering."

Replace Your Blocker Beliefs

"That's a really good thing to do," Bob said. "And now to keep things moving along, our objective this session is to communicate your supportive beliefs directly to your subconscious minds."

"Will this knock out the blocker beliefs?" Ed asked.

"Pretty much," Bob said. "When you get the supportive beliefs in place, powered up, and operational at the subconscious level, that will certainly knock the wind out of the blocker beliefs."

"And we would power them up using the attitude-inoculation challenging question 'why?'" Ed asked.

"Precisely," Bob said. "Remember, to get the best results you need to do this while you're in trance so you can communicate directly with your subconscious mind."

"Any other way we can reduce the power of these old beliefs?" Betty asked.

"When you review them in the 'I used to believe, but that was wrong for me, I now believe' format, draw a line through the old belief as you're saying it. That will symbolically speak to the subconscious mind."

"Oh, I like that," Betty said.

Bob handed out the hypnosis scripts he'd compiled for this session, and said, "Take a few moments to review the blocker beliefs I've included and cross out the ones that don't apply specifically to you. And when you get past those, you'll see I left space for you to write your own. Of course, you can just open your notebook or journal to that page where you prepared yours ahead of time so you're ready when we get to that segment in the script."

Jean looked around and saw that everyone finished, and said, "I have to tell you, I'm excited to finally get to have trance-time with everyone. It's like when John and I go into trance together, I feel a good energy."

171

Everyone nodded.

Betty smiled at Ed and said, "Me too."

"OK, then let's get started," Bob said. "We'll again use the 'blink' induction and I'll use the short version of the body sculpting deepener we've used before."

"It doesn't take us long go into hypnosis, that's for sure," Betty said.

"Then let's start with the question, 'Are you ready to go into hypnosis?'" Bob asked.

Heads nodded.

"And if it's OK with you, will you do what I ask you to do?"

Heads nodded again.

"Always know that should something require your attention while you're in hypnosis, you'll be able to come up and out immediately fully alert and ready to deal with it.

"Let's start by releasing some of the muscle tension and mental distractions by taking a deep breath and as you exhale, feel the tension flow out of your body.

"Again, take a deep refreshing and cleansing breath and exhale. Continue to breathe deeply and comfortably for a little while longer. Focus on your breathing.

"Should you become aware of any sounds or other distractions, simply notice them, let them increase your focus and concentration on this process, and then let them fade away into the background.

"When you read the word 'Breathe' on your hypnosis script, take a deep breath, exhale, and continue reading.

"Take your time with this.

"Whenever you read the word 'BLINK' on your hypnosis script, please blink your eyes and then continue reading.

"Here we go. Want it to happen, expect it to happen, allow it to happen.

"Breathe.
"Five, BLINK.
"Feeling good, focused, anticipating going into trance.
"BLINK.
"No pressure, no rush, slow down.
"BLINK.
"Breathe deeply and exhale. Focus on your breathing.
"Four, BLINK.
"Slowing down.
"BLINK.
"Open to the experience.
"BLINK.
"Going down, deeper down.
"Three, BLINK.
"BLINK.
"Focus on your breathing while you read.
"BLINK.
"Breathe deeply and exhale. In, out, in, out.
"Going slower now.
"Two, BLINK.
"Wonderful feeling going deeper and deeper into trance.
"BLINK.
"Narrow your focus to what you're reading.
"BLINK.
"Breathe deeply and exhale.
"Slower and deeper down.
"One, BLINK.
"Drifting down, feeling good.
"BLINK.
"Focus on the words you're reading, and let the background fade away.
"BLINK.
"Going deeper, deeper down.

"You can blink normally and automatically now.

"Breathe deeply and exhale.

"Whenever you're in trance at any level, you will always be able to read my words to continue through the session and reawaken out of trance when it's time to do so.

"Now imagine that you're at the top of your 10-step staircase.

"At the bottom is the room you created where you communicate with your subconscious mind.

"Each time you move down a step, you'll feel yourself going deeper and deeper into trance. You can step down or gently float down the stairs.

"Ready? Good, now take the handrail and sense its texture and temperature in your hand.

"Ten. Take a deep breath and as you exhale, go down a step.

"Nine. Form your face into the size and shape you want it to be. See it, feel it, own it.

"Eight. Form your jaw and neck into the size and shape you want them to be. See it, feel it, own it.

"Drifting deeper down ... breathe.

"Seven. Form your shoulders and back into the size and shape you want them to be. See it, feel it, own it.

"Six. Form your arms, elbows, forearms, hands, and fingers into the size and shape you want them to be. See it, feel it, own it.

"Floating deeper, deeper down.

"Five. Form your chest into the size and shape you want it to be. See it, feel it, own it.

"Breathe ... Good ... You're doing fine.

"Four. Form your stomach area, waist, and lower back into the size and shape you want it to be. See it, feel it, own it.

"Going down, deeper down.

Replace Your Blocker Beliefs

"Three. Form your hips into the size and shape you want them to be. See it, feel it, own it.

"Two. Form your legs into the size and shape you want them to be. See it, feel it, own it.

"One. Form your ankles, feet, and toes into the size and shape you want them to be. See it, feel it, own it.

"Breathe.

"Go down into the room now. Notice that each time you count yourself down it becomes easier and easier for you to go deeper and deeper into trance.

"Move to the full-length mirrors. The reflection you see is the body your subconscious mind is now guiding you to make in your physical reality.

"Make any adjustments necessary until you see an accurate reflection of your slim, trim, physically fit, trance-formed body. Take a moment to do that now."

Bob paused a minute to give time for any needed adjustments to be made.

"Good. Let's start to change the beliefs that are holding you back to beliefs that will support your slim, trim, physically fit body.

"Look directly into your own eyes in the mirror while you tell your subconscious mind about the beliefs you want to change and what you want to change them to.

"Start with the obsolete belief:

'I used to believe that I had to eat everything on my plate. But that was wrong for me. I now believe that I only want to eat the portions of food I need for nutrition.'

"Now challenge your new belief by asking, 'Why is that important to me?' and answer with emotional power.

"Check to see if the new belief is now strong enough. If not, challenge it again and again until you feel the power. Test it. In your mind, put it into action and see it work for you.

Watch yourself do it from a distance and then when you get a successful outcome and you're ready, mentally step back into your body and do it again.

"Imagine and experience this with your emotions and with as many of your physical senses as you can.

"Notice when it locks in.

"Another obsolete belief to change:

'I used to believe that eating large meals of rich foods was the right thing to do. But that was wrong for me. I now believe my tastes have changed and rich fattening foods now cause my appetite to quickly disappear.'

"Now challenge your new belief by asking, 'Why is that important to me?' and answer with emotional power.

"Check to see if the new belief is now strong enough. If not, challenge it again and again until you feel the power. Test it. In your mind, put it into action and see it work for you. Watch yourself do it from a distance and then when you get a successful outcome and you're ready, mentally step back into your body and do it again.

"Imagine and experience this with your emotions and with as many of your physical senses as you can.

"Notice when it locks in.

"Here's another obsolete belief to change:

'I used to believe that I could only get the good memories I have of my family when I ate the types of food they prepared for me when I was a child. But that was wrong for me. I now believe that I can honor my family and have the good memories by having an occasional special meal with the foods they used to prepare and just take care to eat them in the right portions.'

"Now challenge your new belief by asking, 'Why is that important to me?' and answer with emotional power.

"Check to see if the new belief is now strong enough. If not, challenge it again and again until you feel the power. Test it. In your mind, put it into action and see it work for you. Watch yourself do it from a distance and then when you get a successful outcome and you're ready, mentally step back into your body and do it again.

"Imagine and experience this with your emotions and with as many of your physical senses as you can.

"Notice when it locks in.

"Another obsolete belief to change:

'I used to believe that since my parents were fat that I would be, too. But that was wrong for me. I now know their influence on my weight is minor if any at all. I now believe that I am my own person. I control my own weight, size, and shape. My destiny belongs to me.'

"Now challenge your new belief by asking, 'Why is that important to me?' and answer with emotional power.

"Check to see if the new belief is now strong enough. If not, challenge it again and again until you feel the power. Test it. In your mind, put it into action and see it work for you. Watch yourself do it from a distance and then when you get a successful outcome and you're ready, mentally step back into your body and do it again.

"Imagine and experience this with your emotions and with as many of your physical senses as you can.

"Notice when it locks in.

"Another obsolete belief to change:

'I used to believe that I needed to eat the way I was taught to eat. But that was wrong for me. I now believe that I'm in control of my life, which includes what, when, and how much I chose to eat.'

"Now challenge your new belief by asking, 'Why is that important to me?' and answer with emotional power.

"Check to see if the new belief is now strong enough. If not, challenge it again and again until you feel the power. Test it. In your mind, put it into action and see it work for you. Watch yourself do it from a distance and then when you get a successful outcome and you're ready, mentally step back into your body and do it again.

"Imagine and experience this with your emotions and with as many of your physical senses as you can.

"Notice when it locks in.

"Another obsolete belief to change:

'I used to believe that being fat made me safe. But that was wrong for me. I now believe I am safer and better protected when my body is in good physical condition so that I can take care of myself.'

"Now challenge your new belief by asking, 'Why is that going to keep me safe? What else will I do to keep safe?'"

"Check to see if the new belief is now strong enough. If not, challenge it again and again until you feel the power. Test it. In your mind, put it into action and see it work for you. Watch yourself do it from a distance and then when you get a successful outcome and you're ready, mentally step back into your body and do it again.

"Imagine and experience this with your emotions and with as many of your physical senses as you can.

"Notice when it locks in.

"Another obsolete belief to change:

'I used to believe that whenever I felt anxious or stressed, eating comfort foods would make me calm. But that was wrong for me. I now believe that I can take a deep breath, take a fast short walk and then drink water to make me calm and in control. I have options.'

Replace Your Blocker Beliefs

"Now challenge your new belief by asking, 'Why is that important to me? Where will I walk? Why do I believe I will do this?' and answer with emotional power.

"Check to see if the new belief is now strong enough. If not, challenge it again and again until you feel the power. Test it. In your mind, put it into action and see it work for you. Watch yourself do it from a distance and then when you get a successful outcome and you're ready, mentally step back into your body and do it again.

"Imagine and experience this with your emotions and with as many of your physical senses as you can.

"Notice when it locks in.

"Now let's go through the obsolete beliefs and supportive beliefs you wrote in your journal, notebook, or on these pages.

"'I used to believe _____
But that was wrong for me.
I now believe _____
Why? _____'

"Check to see if the new belief is now strong enough. If not, challenge it again and again until you feel the power. Test it. In your mind, put it into action and see it work for you. Watch yourself do it from a distance and then when you get a successful outcome and you're ready, mentally step back into your body and do it again.

"Imagine and experience this with your emotions and with as many of your physical senses as you can.

"Notice when it locks in.

"'I used to believe _____
But that was wrong for me.
I now believe _____

Why? _____,

"Check to see if the new belief is now strong enough. If not, challenge it again and again until you feel the power. Test it. In your mind, put it into action and see it work for you. Watch yourself do it from a distance and then when you get a successful outcome and you're ready, mentally step back into your body and do it again.

"Imagine and experience this with your emotions and with as many of your physical senses as you can.

"Notice when it locks in.

"'I used to believe _____
But that was wrong for me.
I now believe _____
Why? _____,

"Check to see if the new belief is now strong enough. If not, challenge it again and again until you feel the power. Test it. In your mind, put it into action and see it work for you. Watch yourself do it from a distance and then when you get a successful outcome and you're ready, mentally step back into your body and do it again.

"Imagine and experience this with your emotions and with as many of your physical senses as you can.

"Notice when it locks in.

"Good ... Breathe ...

"You automatically do what is safe, healthy, and necessary for you to achieve and maintain your optimal size and shape.

"You intuitively know what and how much to eat to meet the nutritional needs of your slim, trim, physically fit body.

"You constantly think, act, and eat like the healthy slim, trim, physically fit person you are now and forever.

Replace Your Blocker Beliefs

"It's time now to go to the staircase, reach out, and hold the handrail.

"Notice how you've become comfortable deep in trance. Each time you read yourself into hypnosis, you will find it easier and easier to go into a deeper and deeper level of trance so that you quickly achieve the level that is right for you to communicate effectively with your subconscious mind.

"Whenever you're in trance at any level, you will always be able to read my words to continue through the session and reawaken out of trance when it's time to do so.

"And now, ready.

"Go up to step one in your slim, trim, physically fit body. It's yours now and forever.

"Go up to step two. Feel grateful that your subconscious mind understands and believes in what you want and is now taking action to bring it to physical reality.

"Go up to step three. Notice how your feet, legs, and hips look and move as you go up the stairs.

"Go up to step four. Observe your stomach, waist, lower back. Watch your muscles moving.

"Go up to step five. See your chest moving as you breathe. It's just as you want it to be.

"Go up to step six. Notice your hand on the handrail. Watch your arms move.

"Go up to step seven. See your shoulders and back, muscles toned and moving smoothly.

"Go up to step eight. Observe your jaw and neck. See how they look. They are just as you want them to be.

"Go up to step nine. Notice the smile on your slim, trim face.

"Go up to step ten. Now mentally step back into your body and feel wonderful about the experiences you're having.

"Good, you're doing fine. Breathe.

"You've done well. In a moment, I will count you up and out of trance.

"If you want to intentionally go back to this level of trance in the future, you must agree to bring yourself out of trance when asked to do so.

"Let's start to count up so that you can easily bring yourself up and back into the present time and place.

"One. Coming up now, take a deep breath and come up now.

"Two. Begin to move your body where you are, stretch, and come up even more now.

"Three. Wide awake and back in the present, feeling refreshed, alert, and fully awake.

"Stay where you are for a moment while you increase your alertness. Stretch a little and adjust your posture to help become fully alert."

Jean and Betty were busy writing in their journals to make sure they didn't lose any insights. Ed went to the kitchen and brought back bottles of water for everyone.

"I've got one blocker belief that just isn't cooperating," John said. "It's important because it deals with my feeling of being rejected by my co-workers if I don't join in their daily feasts."

"I think I know what's going on," Bob said. "There's more to with this one than a stubborn blocker belief. Leave it alone for now and we'll deal with it next session."

"Good," John said.

"That was much harder than I thought it would be," Ed said as he settled back in his chair. "I had to really force myself to keep challenging until I got something I could rehearse in my mind and feel strongly that it would work."

"I did, too," Jean said. "But I could tell when my subconscious mind wrapped itself around the new belief."

Replace Your Blocker Beliefs

"Glad to hear that," Bob said. "That's the way it should be."

"What will we be working on next time?" Betty asked.

"The fear center," Bob said.

"I've been waiting for that session," Jean said. "Can you give me the one-sentence overview?"

"Sure," Bob said. "Anything that threatens or causes change can trigger an automatic brain function that will do everything in its exceptionally powerful arsenal to stop the threat and reverse the change."

"Everything we're doing here is about change," Jean said.

"And that's why you must harness the power of this fear center," Bob said. "If you don't get it working for you, it will fight hard to stop your ability to change your weight, size, and shape.

"We seem to be moving along OK now," John said. "It doesn't seem to be interfering yet."

"That's because," Bob said, "you've already started harnessing its power from the first time you got your subconscious minds to believe that the slim, trim body you are imagining is your true body and any actions that would threaten it must be stopped."

"You got it on our side from the very beginning?" Jean asked.

"Yes," Bob said. "I had to or you could have hit a plateau. Your fear center, which also operates at the subconscious level, is now buying into that image and starting to protect it. But there is still a lot more we need to do and do quickly in this area."

"Is there anything we need to do to prepare for the session?" Jean asked.

"No," Bob said. "Just bring your fears."

"Funny," Ed said.

"I know we've got to stop for this session," Betty said. "But can we get back together tomorrow about this same time?"

Everyone agreed, and the group reluctantly broke up for the evening.

Chapter 12 Harness Your Fears

The next day after everyone settled back into their familiar chairs, Bob said. "If everyone's ready, let's jump back into our discussion about the fear center."

"I know we touched on this before when we first met and a little more yesterday," Ed said, "but can we take this from the beginning?"

"Good idea," Bob said. "We all have these brain structures called the amygdalae. There are two of them. Among other things, one of their primary functions is to help us survive by alerting us and reacting to danger. These are your fear centers."

"That doesn't sound too bad," Ed said.

"Most of the time it's a good thing," Bob said. "It's continually monitoring your internal and external environments for anything that might threaten you. If it notices anything it remembers as dangerous or sees anything different that could pose a threat, it becomes hyper-vigilant and ready to react."

"Like automatically hitting the brakes when something jumps in front of you," Ed said.

"That's a good example," Bob said.

"Everything so far seems in order," Ed said. "How does this affect our weight-control efforts?"

"One of the ways the fear center operates is by detecting change," Bob said. "Change is usually regarded as a threat. It is the fear of the unknown that causes it to react. Sometimes we're totally unaware that we resisted a change and sometimes we are aware but don't know why we responded as we did."

"We talked about this earlier," Ed said. "But could the fear center cause people to shoot down new ideas before they even know what they're about?"

"That's part of it," Bob said. "The greater the change, the greater the resistance."

"We're all making some pretty big changes," Jean said.

"Yes, you are," Bob said. "When your fear center senses a change in your eating patterns such as reducing how much you eat, or what you're eating, how much you're exercising, a change in lifestyle, or really any change for that matter, it could interpret those changes as threats and if so, it would automatically attempt to stop them from taking place."

"That's pretty intense," John said. "But wouldn't we know?"

"Very often you would," Bob said. "You could, for example, be faced with a choice of eating something healthy but new, or something unhealthy, but familiar. The fear center doesn't think. It just reacts. It will do what it can to get you to choose the familiar."

"Does that mean the changes we tried in the past to drop a few pounds could have fallen victim to this fear center?" Jean asked.

"Possibly," Bob said. "There are a lot of high-quality weight control programs available that are effective so long as you continue to make rigorous conscious efforts to carry out the directions. But most will fail in the long run if you don't win the mental game at the subconscious level as well. Helping you win the mental game is really what our sessions are all about."

"Now that's an interesting thought," John said. "This could mean that we might have been on the right track with our previous efforts but then this fear center stopped us without our even knowing it."

"Again entirely possible," Bob said. "I would also toss in body image issues, ineffective stress coping mechanisms, weak motivators, and blocker beliefs. But even with those taken care of as you're now doing, when it comes to weight control, your fear center would rather keep you in a known fat state than face an unknown state posed by change. To it, change is scary."

"Why fat?" John asked.

"Remember our discussion about the starvation reflex?" Bob asked.

"Yeah," John said. "The brain thinks we're going into a famine and stores fat."

"Ah," Jean said, "because, without fat to carry us through the famine, we'll die."

"So your survival mechanisms like to store fat," Bob said.

"That explains a lot," Jean said.

"This fear center is also in a constant state of learning," Bob said. "It has to continually evaluate new threats. That's how it helps you survive. But sometimes it gets it wrong as happens when you do normal types of things to change your body's weight, size, and shape."

"So what do we do?" Ed asked.

"For weight-control purposes, you'll have to learn how to harness its power and how to retrain it so that it doesn't sabotage your weight-control efforts," Bob said.

"I'm ready. How do we do that?" Ed asked.

"There are two ways to do this," Bob said. "You've already started doing the first one, which is to redirect the threat factor to something you believe you already have that would be put in jeopardy.

"Our slim, trim bodies," Betty said.

"I get it," Ed said. "We imagined already having it and owning it and now our subconscious mind believes it's real."

"How do you think your fear center will react if it perceives a threat that you might lose it?" Bob asked.

"If we believe it's real at the subconscious level, then the fear center will actually help us keep it?" Ed asked. "And that's why you had us use hypnosis to convince the subconscious mind that the bodies we want are our true bodies?"

"Yes," Bob said. "You had to get the image so clear and ingrained that you could instantly call it up into your conscious minds. Once you were able to do that, you automatically put the fear center on your side."

"You said two ways," Ed said.

"The second way," Bob said, "is to retrain the fear center to become aware of what it perceives as a threat is really not a threat. The easiest way is to muster up the courage to do the behavior and show there are no ill effects. That way the fear center learns that the things you're doing to make changes to your body are not threats and the change to your body itself is not a threat."

"How do we do that?" Betty asked. "Can you give me an example?"

"OK," Bob said. "Let's make this easy by combining the two methods. Can you conjure up the feeling of fear or worry?"

"I guess so," Betty said.

"Imagine a healthy food and a fattening food," Bob said. "Now say the words to yourself, 'I'm afraid to eat the fattening food because it would put my slim and trim body at risk.' And when you imagine losing your slim and trim body, feel the fear or worry associated with making the wrong choice."

"Oh, that hit me hard," Betty said.

"Me, too," Jean said.

"Now let's teach your fear center that eating healthy foods is not going to hurt you," Bob said. "Go back and imagine the same situation of feeling the fear associated with making the wrong choice. Now make the right choice and imagine eating the healthy food. Notice how good that feels."

"That felt nice," Betty said.

Harness Your Fears

"With this process," Bob said, "you first harnessed the power of the fear center by shifting the threat from the new healthy food to the familiar fattening food. At the same time, by pushing through and imagining eating the better choice, your fear center learned that the new healthy food is not threatening and it's OK to eat it. It now becomes the familiar non-threatening choice."

"Do another example, please," Ed said.

"Sure," Bob said. "Ask yourself, 'do I eat the whole piece of pie and suffer the loss of my slim, trim body or do I protect it by only taking a bite or two of the pie?' At this point get into the feeling of fear. And this is critically important for this to work, you must actually be afraid of losing your slim, trim body. Feel the fear and then redirect and associate it with eating the whole piece."

"Got it," Ed said. "I look at something I might want to eat but I know would do harm to the body I'm building. I put the fear factor on it by saying 'I'm afraid of what will happen if I eat that,' and at the same time feel the fear of losing the body I want."

"Oh, yeah," John said. "That ties the fear to the fattening food and the risk of losing our slim, trim bodies."

"And at the same time we're training the fear center not to fear eating something nutritious," Jean said.

"And," Bob said, "it doesn't always have to do with food."

"What do you mean?" Betty asked.

"You could be making a choice about things you want to do," Bob said. "One choice would get you up and moving around like going to an event or taking a walk and the other would have you become physically inactive like watching TV."

"We need to be alert to all the choices we make that could impact our bodies," Ed said.

"Just make and carry out the right choice so you let the fear center learn that it didn't harm you," Bob said. "And at the same time reinforce how making the wrong choice threatens the survival of your healthy body."

"I've been complimented on the progress I'm making and would be embarrassed to lose it now. Would fear of embarrassment work as well?"

"Even better," Bob said. "With this added, you've compounded the negative consequences of making wrong decisions regarding your weight, size, and shape goals."

"Do we need to go into trance for this to work?" Betty asked.

"Very good question," Bob said. "Emotional learning, especially when the fear emotion is involved and is strong, usually only takes one exposure for the learning to be permanent at the subconscious level.

"To answer your question then, by imagining the situation and actually feeling the fear, you automatically experienced a micro-trance and so using a formal trance process isn't always necessary."

"If we wanted to use a full trance, it would be OK?" Betty asked.

"Absolutely," Bob said. "We'll be doing that here in a few minutes. It makes sense to go through this harnessing and training process using a formal trance until you can recognize when your fear shifts and is redirected to the prospect of losing the body your subconscious believes is the true you."

"Thank you," Betty said. "Once we know what the shift feels like, then we can use the micro-trance anywhere we need to like when we're looking at menus or at the bakery."

"But how would we know for sure if it worked?" Ed asked.

Harness Your Fears

"Let's take the pie example," Bob said. "Next time you're at the grocery store, go smell the pies and see what happens."

"If the pie scares me that means it worked?" Ed asked.

"Well, I'm not sure you would be afraid of the pie," Bob said. "But I am sure that you would sense some alarm about the damage the pie would do to your weight, size, and shape goals if you ate the whole thing."

"Now that you've got a really good understanding of the process, let's take a quick look at some of the things that can trigger the fear center related to food."

Bob handed out a list and said, "Just like the other lists I've given you, this is only a sampling of ideas that will help stimulate your thinking about your own fears related to your goals.

"Just fill in the blank when you say, 'I overeat because of my fear of…'

- offending or upsetting someone if I turn down the food they offer
- being rejected or disapproved of if I don't join in and eat all the food they're eating
- feeling vulnerable if I don't have fat as body armor
- being alone
- strong emotions aimed at me like anger, shame, disgust, or guilt
- feeling depressed, sad, hopeless, or self-pity
- emotional conflicts within me that make me want to eat comfort foods
- not getting enough to eat

"Can anyone pick one or two that hit home?" Bob asked.

"The first two on the list are mine," Betty said.

"Me, too," John said.

"Can you go through some examples of how we could deal with these?" Ed asked.

"Let's use the format at the bottom of the list I gave you so all we have to do is fill in the blanks," Bob said.

I used to overeat because of my fear of _____
But now I'm more afraid of losing my slim, trim body I'm working so hard to get and keep.
I now believe _____
Why? _____

"This looks familiar to the way we dealt with our obsolete beliefs," John said.

"Very close," Bob said. "Here you're going to shift the fear from the thing that you're currently afraid of to being more afraid of losing you slim, trim body that you've worked so hard to get."

"What if the problem isn't overeating, but rather it's with what I'm eating?" John asked. "Like comfort food or junk food."

"You can eat comfort food and even junk food if you eat it in the right portions," Bob said. "It's when you overeat whatever food you're eating, that's when you into trouble."

"Yeah," John said. "I can see that. So we only need to think about the overeating part."

"That's right," Bob said.

"Can you give me a quick example redirecting the fear?" Ed asked.

"Sure," Bob said. "I'll do the first one on the list."

"Good," John said. "I need that one."

"I do too," Betty said.

"OK, here goes," Bob said. "I used to overeat because of my fear of offending my friends if I turn down the food they offer. But now I'm more afraid of losing my slim, trim body I'm working so hard to get and keep." Bob said.

"Got it," Ed said.

"So you're making one fear scarier than the other," John said.

"Yes," Bob said. "And we're putting the 'overeating' in the past tense to signal to your subconscious mind that you no longer want that. You're also using 'but' as an eraser."

"An eraser?" Ed asked.

"The word 'but' erases everything that was said in front of it," Bob said. "For example, suppose I said, 'you're doing a good job, but.'"

"Ouch," Ed said. "So much for the 'good job.' It went away as soon as you said 'but.'"

"Next," Bob said, "It's time to put a new belief in place to train your fear centers that you have alternatives that won't threaten your survival."

"And I see in the format that we challenge them to lock them in place as attitudes," Betty said.

"Exactly," Bob said. "So let's take an example of the one I started earlier of being afraid of offending your friends if you turn down food they're offering you. Let's use the format and fill in the blanks.

"I used to overeat because of my fear of offending my friends if I turn down food they offer me. But now I'm more afraid of losing my slim, trim body I'm working so hard to get and keep. I now believe my friends will accept my decision when I let them know about my goals and my fears. Why? And then continue the challenges as needed to identify your motivators and lock them in place as you've done many times before."

"Could you do an example with my experience?" Jean asked.

"Sure," Bob said. "Let's use the standard format to see how it can work for you."

"Good," she said.

"I used to overeat because of my fear of being vulnerable without my fat as body armor. But now I'm more afraid of losing my slim, trim body I'm working so hard to get and keep. I now believe that being physically fit gives me better body armor and greater safety."

"I could really feel that," Jean said. "Thank you."

"I think we all agree with that as well," Ed said. "It really does make you realize that it is fear that's stopping you from making the right choices."

"And," John added, "with the rest of the format we have a way to teach the fear center that there is an option so our fear centers won't react against what we want."

"Is this an obsolete fear like we had obsolete beliefs?" Betty asked.

"The fear is obsolete because it's not serving your best interest," Bob said. "But, at this time, the subconscious mind might not accept a suggestion based on the premise that the fear is no longer valid or that you no longer have that fear when at the onset it senses at the conscious and subconscious levels you do still feel the fear.

"Emotions are so fully integrated with everything at the subconscious level and are such a powerhouse of influence that they have to be handled a little differently than beliefs."

"Now I understand why I couldn't get my fear of offending my coworkers to work with the blocker belief format," John said.

"Does that mean we keep the fear?" Betty asked.

"Only until your fear center experiences a couple successful outcomes with your new belief," Bob said. "At that time the old fear will weaken and become only a cautionary memory rather than a controlling obstructive fear."

"Can we just imagine putting our new belief into use like we did with the blocker beliefs and get the same result?" John asked.

"Yes," Bob said. "You'll definitely want to rehearse the new belief being successful while in trance to the point that it dominates your feelings whenever the fear trigger shows up."

"And we'd challenge the heck out of the new belief to make sure it's powered up and locked in place," Ed said.

"Absolutely," Bob said. "Like you've done before, you'll want to rehearse it first by watching yourself carry out the new belief at a distance and then when you have a successful outcome and you're ready you can mentally step back into your body and do it again. You'll know when it locks in."

"How far is a distance?" Ed asked.

"If it's emotionally tough or scary, make it a long distance, and then as your comfort level increases, you can gradually bring it closer with each round of practice," Bob said. "If it's non-threatening, the distance could be as close as seeing yourself in the mirrors."

"That really is powerful," Jean said. "It was so clear to me when the shift was made with the motivators and the blocker beliefs."

"Let me go through a couple more examples so we can all feel comfortable with this structure," Bob said.

"Could you do one with my fear of being rejected by my friends again?" Betty asked. "I know we just did it, but I didn't get it all down."

"Sure," Bob said. "Let me broaden the scope to include other people such as family or coworkers."

"Great," Betty said.

"I used to overeat because of my fear of being rejected or disapproved of by people I care about when I turn down food they offer. But now I'm more afraid of losing my slim, trim body I'm working so hard to get and keep. I now believe that it's more about the people than about the food and they will understand and accept my decision when they learn about my goals and fears."

"That's really good," Betty said. "Thank you."

"Let's do an example about being lonely," Bob said.

"I used to overeat because of my fear of feeling lonely. But now I'm more afraid of losing my slim, trim body I'm working so hard to get and keep. I now believe that I can be alone and not be lonely by using this opportunity to do the things I enjoy doing by myself."

"Does everyone get the pattern?" Bob asked.

Heads nodded in agreement.

"So here's what we'll do then," Bob said. "Take a few minutes to identify your top three fears and write them in your journals or notebooks using this pattern."

I used to overeat because of my fear of _____

But now I'm more afraid of losing my slim, trim body I'm working so hard to get and keep.

I now believe _____

Why? _____

Bob paused while they wrote out their fears and new beliefs.

Ed asked, "Are there other fears operating at the subconscious level that we could find if we used the same process we did to find hidden motivators and hidden blocker beliefs?"

"You certainly could," Bob said. "In fact, why don't we add that question at the end of this sequence while you're already in trance? For example, after you've completed the work with the fears you already know about in front of the mirrors, I'll ask you to move over to your books on the desk to write the question, 'What else am I afraid of that would interfere with the body I'm forming?'"

"That would sure save a step," Betty said.

"You'll want to bring those newly uncovered fears back to your conscious level so you can develop your new beliefs and get the wording the way you want it," Bob said. "Then you can go back into trance to redirect the fears directly with your subconscious minds.

"If you want to prepare ahead of time, you could also reinforce any of the previous work you've done."

"I didn't think about combining them into one session," John said.

"Just don't overload yourself," Bob said. "Any more than five of any type is pushing the limits."

"Any other questions?" Bob asked.

Heads shook.

"OK then," Bob said, "Are you ready to go into hypnosis to deal with these fears?"

Heads nodded enthusiastically, and Ed said, "Lead the way. We're ready."

"And if it's OK with you, will you do what I ask you to do?"

Heads nodded again.

"Always know that should something require your attention while you're in hypnosis, you'll be able to come up and out immediately fully alert and ready to deal with it.

"Let's start by releasing some of the muscle tension and mental distractions by taking a deep breath, and as you exhale feel the tension flow out of your body.

"Again, take a deep refreshing and cleansing breath and exhale. Continue to breathe deeply and comfortably for a little while longer. Focus on your breathing.

"Should you become aware of any sounds or other distractions, simply notice them, let them increase your focus and concentration on this process, and then let them fade away into the background.

"When you read the word 'Breathe' on your hypnosis script, take a deep breath, exhale, and continue reading.

"Take your time with this.

"Whenever you read the word 'BLINK' on your hypnosis script, please blink your eyes and then continue reading.

"Here we go. Want it to happen, expect it to happen, allow it to happen.

"Breathe.

"Five, BLINK.

"Feeling good, focused, anticipating going into trance.

"BLINK.

"No pressure, no rush, slow down.

"BLINK.

"Breathe deeply and exhale. Focus on your breathing.

"Four, BLINK.

"Slowing down.

"BLINK.

"Open to the experience.

"BLINK.

"Going down, deeper down.

"Three, BLINK.

"BLINK.

"Focus on your breathing while you read.

"BLINK.

"Breathe deeply and exhale. In, out, in, out.

"Going slower now.

"Two, BLINK.

"Wonderful feeling going deeper and deeper into trance.

"BLINK.

"Narrow your focus to what you're reading.

"BLINK.

"Breathe deeply and exhale.

"Slower and deeper down.

"One, BLINK.

"Drifting down, feeling good.

"BLINK.

"Focus on the words you're reading, and let the background fade away.

"BLINK.

"Going deeper, deeper down.

"You can blink normally and automatically now.

"Breathe deeply and exhale.

"Whenever you're in trance at any level, you will always be able to read my words to continue through the session and reawaken out of trance when it's time to do so.

"Now imagine that you're at the top of your 10-step staircase.

"At the bottom is the room you created where you communicate with your subconscious mind.

"Each time you move down a step, you'll feel yourself going deeper and deeper into trance. You can step down or gently float down the stairs.

"Ready? Good, now take the handrail and sense its texture and temperature in your hand.

"Ten. Take a deep breath and as you exhale, go down a step.

Trance Formed Body

"Nine. Form your face into the size and shape you want it to be. See it, feel it, own it.

"Eight. Form your jaw and neck into the size and shape you want them to be. See it, feel it, own it.

"Drifting deeper down ... breathe.

"Seven. Form your shoulders and back into the size and shape you want them to be. See it, feel it, own it.

"Six. Form your arms, elbows, forearms, hands, and fingers into the size and shape you want them to be. See it, feel it, own it.

"Floating deeper, deeper down.

"Five. Form your chest into the size and shape you want it to be. See it, feel it, own it.

"Breathe ... Good ... You're doing fine.

"Four. Form your stomach area, waist, and lower back into the size and shape you want it to be. See it, feel it, own it.

"Going down, deeper down.

"Three. Form your hips into the size and shape you want them to be. See it, feel it, own it.

"Two. Form your legs into the size and shape you want them to be. See it, feel it, own it.

"One. Form your ankles, feet, and toes into the size and shape you want them to be. See it, feel it, own it.

"Breathe.

"Go down into the room now. Notice that each time you count yourself down, it becomes easier and easier for you to go deeper and deeper into trance.

"Move to the full-length mirrors. The reflection you see is the body your subconscious mind is now guiding you to make in your physical reality.

"Make any adjustments necessary until you see an accurate reflection of your slim, trim, physically fit, trance-formed body. Take a moment to do that now.

Harness Your Fears

"Good. Let's start to redirect the fears that are holding you back and embed new beliefs that will support your slim, trim, physically fit body.

"Look directly into your own eyes in the mirror while you tell your subconscious mind how you are adjusting and training your fear center to respond more appropriately to your needs.

"'I used to overeat because of my fear of _____
But now I'm more afraid of losing my slim, trim body I'm working so hard to get and keep.
    I now believe _____
    Why? _____,

"Check to see if the new belief is now strong enough. If not, challenge it again and again until you feel the power. Test it. In your mind, put it into action and see it work for you. Watch yourself do it from a distance and then when you get a successful outcome and you're ready, mentally step back into your body and do it again.

"Imagine and experience this with your emotions and with as many of your physical senses as you can.

"Notice when it locks in.

"'I used to overeat because of my fear of _____
But now I'm more afraid of losing my slim, trim body I'm working so hard to get and keep.
    I now believe _____
    Why? _____,

"Check to see if the new belief is now strong enough. If not, challenge it again and again until you feel the power. Test it. In your mind, put it into action and see it work for you. Watch yourself do it from a distance and then when you get a successful outcome and you're ready, mentally step back into your body and do it again.

"Imagine and experience this with your emotions and with as many of your physical senses as you can.

"Notice when it locks in.

"'I used to overeat because of my fear of _____
But now I'm more afraid of losing my slim, trim body I'm working so hard to get and keep.
I now believe _____
Why? _____,'

"Check to see if the new belief is now strong enough. If not, challenge it again and again until you feel the power. Test it. In your mind, put it into action and see it work for you. Watch yourself do it from a distance and then when you get a successful outcome and you're ready, mentally step back into your body and do it again.

"Imagine and experience this with your emotions and with as many of your physical senses as you can.

"Notice when it locks in.

"Good ... Breathe ...

"Now move to your book on the tall table. Open it and write your question, 'what else am I afraid of that could interfere with the slim, trim, physically fit body I'm creating?'

"Take a minute to go deep into your subconscious mind to find any other fears that interfere with achieving your weight, size, and shape goals. Write any responses in your book. When you're finished, close the book and leave it on the table. You'll remember what you wrote when you come out of trance."

Bob paused for a minute and then said, "It's time now to go to the staircase, reach out, and hold the handrail.

Harness Your Fears

"You automatically do what is safe, healthy, and necessary for you to maintain your optimal size and shape.

"You intuitively know what and how much to eat to meet the nutritional needs for your slim, trim, physically fit body.

"You constantly think, act, and eat like the healthy slim, trim, physically fit person you are now and forever.

"Whenever you're in trance at any level, you will always be able to read my words to continue through the session and reawaken out of trance when it's time to do so.

"And now, ready.

"Go up to step one in your slim, trim, physically fit body. It's yours now and forever.

"Go up to step two. Feel grateful that your subconscious mind understands and believes in what you want and is now taking action to bring it to physical reality.

"Go up to step three. Notice how your feet, legs, and hips look and move as you go up the stairs.

"Go up to step four. Observe your stomach, waist, lower back. Watch your muscles moving.

"Go up to step five. See your chest moving as you breathe. It's just as you want it to be.

"Go up to step six. Notice your hand on the handrail. Watch your arms move.

"Go up to step seven. See your shoulders and back, muscles toned and moving smoothly.

"Go up to step eight. Observe your jaw and neck. See how they look. They are just as you want them to be.

"Go up to step nine. Notice the smile on your slim, trim face.

"Go up to step ten. Now mentally step back into your body and feel wonderful about the experiences you're having.

"Good, you're doing fine. Breathe.

"You've done well. In a moment, I will count you up and out of trance.

"If you want to intentionally go back to this level of trance in the future, you must agree to bring yourself out of trance when asked to do so.

"Let's start to count up so that you can easily bring yourself up and back into the present time and place.

"One. Coming up now, take a deep breath and come up now.

"Two. Begin to move your body where you are, stretch, and come up even more now.

"Three. Wide awake and back in the present, feeling refreshed, alert, and fully awake.

"Stay where you are for a moment while you increase your alertness. Stretch a little and adjust your posture to help become fully alert."

Everyone smiled with a sense of accomplishment and confidence washing over them.

"OK," Jean said. "I was at wit's end trying to figure out why John and I couldn't do what we knew we had to do, and now I know why. But now I'm wondering why my fear center didn't stop me from doing what we're now doing?"

"I think I know the answer to that," Ed said.

"Please enlighten," John chuckled but with a tone of seriousness.

"Everything we did," Ed said, "had a basis of pure logic and common sense to it. So my guess is that the fear center didn't sense a threat. Am I right, Dr. Bob?"

"I think you've given a very good explanation of what we been doing," Bob said.

"What do we do next?" Betty asked.

Harness Your Fears

"Well, first of all," Bob said, "you've got your work cut out for you now, organizing and implementing what you've discovered so far."

Heads nodded.

"On top of that and in preparation for our next session, I want you to think about this," Bob said. "I gave you a formula, but every answer came from within you."

Heads nodded again.

"Now here is the big one. Your mind and body already know how to build or restore the slim, trim, physically fit person you want to be. You just have to get the message through to your subconscious mind that this is what you want."

"Before we learned hypnosis, getting that message through was all but impossible," John said.

"Yeah, I know," Bob said. "Dale Carnegie, a great trainer and public speaker, said that 'if you want to be enthusiastic, act enthusiastic.' Eventually, your subconscious mind will get the message that it's supposed to be enthusiastic and wham, you are."

"That's why you keep telling us to think thin, see the thin person in you, feed the thin person, focus on your thin," Ed said.

"Yes," Bob said. "Except for the magnitude and complexity of what you're trying to do, it's not very different. 'If you want to be slim and trim, act slim and trim. Feed the thin person and that's who will emerge. Yes, Ed, focus on your thin."

"OK," Jean said. "That was funny. True, but funny."

"What's on the agenda for our next session?" Ed asked.

"Without spoiling the surprise, let me just say that the next time we get together we're going to learn one of the most wonderful and powerful hypnotic meditations, soaking up the colors of the rainbow to awaken and strengthen core characteristics, beliefs, values, and other internal resources that will support you on your lifelong fun adventures in your slim, trim, physically fit body."

"This sounds like the icing on the cake," Betty asked.

Bob laughed and then said, "It is. This will help fortify and seal in the flavor."

"I'm not even going to ask," Ed said.

"Betty," Bob said, "would you do the honors again and coordinate schedules for our next encounter?"

"Be delighted."

Chapter 13 Access Your Internal Resources

Everyone, including Dr. Bob, arrived early for the session. They got their refreshments and took their familiar seats.

"Glad to see everyone is as excited as I am about this session," Bob said.

"We're ready," John said. "I'm really fascinated about how we're going to use colors to stimulate our internal strengths."

"Then let's jump right in," Bob said. "We're going to use a brilliant white full-spectrum light shining through a crystal prism to create the seven colors of the rainbows. I like to use these colors because most people already have positive meanings and good feelings associated with them."

"I know that different colors bring out different emotions in me," Jean said.

"In our everyday lives, we associate colors with different mental, emotional, and physical sensations," Bob said. "That's one reason different colors with different meanings affect us in different ways."

"My favorite color is yellow," Betty said. "When I see it, I feel happy. Ed says it gives me a sunny disposition. Yellow just fills me with joy."

"And now ladies and gentleman," Ed said waving his arms and pointing toward the kitchen, "that explains why her kitchen is yellow, her aprons are yellow, and everything else as far as the eye can see is yellow. She is one happy camper, and I love that about her."

"Will we feel these colors in trance?" Betty asked.

"Good question," Bob said. "There is a very rare condition in which people actually feel, hear, and taste colors. But again, that's not what we're going for here. Just like you do with the color yellow, most all people give meaning to colors, and most all people experience and respond to different colors in different ways."

"I'm thinking just knowing the meanings could cause changes," John said. "Would that be like responding the way we did when we thought about the pickle?"

"To a very large extent, yes," Bob said. "What kind of positive things come to mind when you think about the color red?"

"Passion," Jean said. "Red dress."

"Courage comes to mind," Ed said.

"Is that a color you would associate with hot or cold?" Bob asked.

"Hot," John said.

"What does hot temperature feel like physically?" Bob asked.

"Standing close to a fireplace or stepping down into a hot tub," John said.

"So now you have meanings, emotions, and a temperature associated with this color," Bob said. "Just imagine for a moment that you can feel the heat flowing up through your body fueling your passion to achieve your weight, size, and shape goals. Sense the courage you feel surging through your body to continue to move forward no matter what obstacle steps in your way."

"That was great," Jean said. "We're going to do that with all the different colors?"

"Yes," Bob said. "You already have many sensations attached to each of these colors and even with the white light. Our focus in trance will be to bring out the positive effects that can help you with your size and shape goals."

"Even the light of day will be helping us?" John asked.

Bob smiled and nodded.

"I heard something about how we need to have full-spectrum light," Jean said.

"That's because some people who don't have a certain amount of full-spectrum or natural light can become depressed," John said. "What's that called?"

"Seasonal affective disorder or SAD," Bob said. "It's often treated by exposing the person to full-spectrum light for a pre-defined amount of time each day."

"So colors have energy that can move through our bodies?" Betty asked.

"Oh, I know about this from my work in the lab," John said. "Colors have different vibrational frequencies and wavelengths. Higher on the light spectrum at a faster vibration you have x-rays that can take pictures of the inside your body."

"Even with the color spectrum we can see," Bob said, "we can let our imaginations carry this energy throughout our bodies and into every cell. This imagery helps stimulate the mental, emotional, and physical sensations we get with each color."

"Just like we did with the color red?" Jean asked.

"Yes," Bob said. "And again, I'll guide you through the more common positive meanings people have with these colors. You can then add any special meaning each color has for you personally."

"Like yellow does for me," Betty said.

"Yes," Bob said. "Yellow helps you access resources you already have."

"Is that like knowing how to use these tools like we talked about last time?" Jean asked.

"It is and it's more," Bob said. "Along with the tools you learned, you also have a number of characteristics, beliefs, values, and other internal resources that can be accessed to guide and support you. What we're going to do is call up and create a greater awareness of them. You'll do that in a way that will let you sense them mentally, physically, and emotionally."

With excitement in her voice, Betty said, "The door, the door. I figured it out. The colors are behind the door."

"Yes, they are," Bob said. "Moving on then. For this fascinating journey, you'll use the same trance induction and deepening process that we've been using to make it easy for you to go deeper into trance.

"Once in your hypnosis imagery room at the bottom of the stairs, you'll check the mirrors, dress for the occasion, and then you'll open the door. On the other side of the door, you'll find a room with a very large crystal prism.

"In this room, a brilliant white light shines down from above at an angle that causes the crystal to activate and energize a rainbow of colors around the room."

"I've got all sorts of crystal prisms in my store that make the walls dance with color," Jean said.

"Isn't that an awesome thing to see?" Bob asked.

"Truly awesome," Jean said. "And I get to see it almost every day."

"That's great," Bob said. "After we finish this session, every time you see the colors you'll be reminded of your personal strengths."

"Jean," Betty said. "I'll be stopping by your store tomorrow to get one for Ed and me."

"And," Bob said, "if you want something to remind you, anything with the colors will do nicely."

"Good," Ed said.

"For our session," Bob said, "when the white light hits this exceptionally large crystal, it will split the light so that each, energy-filled color shines separately in a different part of the room."

Access Your Internal Resources

"And that's how we can experience the sensations and meanings of each color by itself," Jean said.

"Yes," Bob said. "I've also included a place in the script where you can explore and discover any special meaning each of the colors may have for you that will serve you in your quest for the body you want."

"Start now," Betty said. "I'm ready."

"Everyone else ready to go into trance?" Bob asked.

Heads nodded and people shifted in their seats to get into a more comfortable position.

"And if it meets with your approval, will you do what I ask you to do?"

Heads nodded again.

"Good," Bob said. "As always, know that should something require your attention while you're in hypnosis, you'll be able to come up and out immediately, fully alert and ready to deal with it.

"Let's start by releasing some of the muscle tension and mental distractions by taking a deep breath and as you exhale feel the tension flow out of your body.

"Again, take a deep refreshing and cleansing breath and exhale. Continue to breathe deeply and comfortably for a little while longer. Focus on your breathing.

"Should you become aware of any sounds or other distractions, simply notice them, let them increase your focus and concentration on this process, and then let them fade away into the background.

"When you read the word 'Breathe' on your hypnosis script take a deep breath, exhale, and continue reading.

"Take your time with this.

"Whenever you read the word 'BLINK' on your hypnosis script, please blink your eyes and then continue reading.

"Here we go. Want it to happen, expect it to happen, allow it to happen.

"Breathe.

"Five, BLINK.

"Feeling good, focused, anticipating going into trance.

"BLINK.

"No pressure, no rush, slow down.

"BLINK.

"Breathe deeply and exhale. Focus on your breathing.

"Four, BLINK.

"Slowing down.

"BLINK.

"Open to the experience.

"BLINK.

"Going down, deeper down.

"Three, BLINK.

"BLINK.

"Focus on your breathing while you read.

"BLINK.

"Breathe deeply and exhale. In, out, in, out.

"Going slower now.

"Two, BLINK.

"Wonderful feeling going deeper and deeper into trance.

"BLINK.

"Narrow your focus to what you're reading.

"BLINK.

"Breathe deeply and exhale.

"Slower and deeper down.

"One, BLINK.

"Drifting down, feeling good.

"BLINK.

"Focus on the words you're reading, and let the background fade away.

"BLINK.

"Going deeper, deeper down.

"You can blink normally and automatically now.

"Breathe deeply and exhale.

"Whenever you're trance at any level, you will always be able to read my words to continue through the session and reawaken out of trance when it's time to do so.

Now imagine that you're at the top of your 10-step staircase.

"At the bottom is the room you created where you communicate with your subconscious mind.

"Each time you move down a step, you'll feel yourself going deeper and deeper into trance. You can step down or gently float down the stairs.

"Ready? Good, now take the handrail and sense its texture and temperature in your hand.

"Ten. Take a deep breath and as you exhale, go down a step.

"Nine. Form your face into the size and shape you want it to be. See it, feel it, own it.

"Eight. Form your jaw and neck into the size and shape you want them to be. See it, feel it, own it.

"Drifting deeper down ... breathe.

"Seven. Form your shoulders and back into the size and shape you want them to be. See it, feel it, own it.

"Six. Form your arms, elbows, forearms, hands, and fingers into the size and shape you want them to be. See it, feel it, own it.

"Floating deeper, deeper down.

"Five. Form your chest into the size and shape you want it to be. See it, feel it, own it.

"Breathe ... Good ... You're doing fine.

"Four. Form your stomach area, waist, and lower back into the size and shape you want it to be. See it, feel it, own it.

"Going down, deeper down.

"Three. Form your hips into the size and shape you want them to be. See it, feel it, own it.

"Two. Form your legs into the size and shape you want them to be. See it, feel it, own it.

"One. Form your ankles, feet, and toes into the size and shape you want them to be. See it, feel it, own it.

"Breathe.

"Go down into the room now. Notice that each time you count yourself down, it becomes easier and easier for you to go deeper and deeper into trance.

"Move to the full-length mirrors. The reflection you see is the body your subconscious mind is now guiding you to make in your physical reality.

"Make any adjustments necessary until you see an accurate reflection of your slim, trim, physically fit, trance-formed body. Take a moment to do that now.

"Good, now go to your open closet to select and change into the clothes that you intuitively know will be comfortable for this journey through the colors of the rainbow. Once you begin, you can still instantly change clothes as you like just by thinking about what you want to wear.

"Move over to the door, take a deep breath, and as you exhale, open it wide.

"Imagine that behind the door is a room with a very large crystal prism. A brilliant white light shines down from above causing the crystal to activate and energize a rainbow of colors around the room.

"Each energy-filled color shines separately in a different part of the room from floor to ceiling.

Access Your Internal Resources

"In a moment you will move through the colors, and as you enter each color, sense its energy and be open to the positive qualities it stimulates within you.

"Step into the room and take a deep breath, and as you exhale move over to the part of the room where the red band of light shines brightest.

"As you move into the clear red light energy, feel yourself go deeper and deeper into trance.

"Notice this slow vibrating earthly red energy flowing through your entire body.

"Feel the power of the red energy ignite your passion and courage to do what you know you must do to quickly and safely get and keep the body you want and deserve.

"Sense the red energy restoring youthful vitality to your slim, trim, physically fit, trance-formed body.

"Breathe ...

"Become aware now of any personal meaning the color red has for you. How can that help you achieve your weight, size, and shape goals?"

Bob paused for a minute and then continued.

"Breathe ... Good ...

"Next to the red light is a bright orange band of light.

"Move into the clear orange light energy and go deeper down into trance.

"Sense the orange energy flowing through every part of your slim, trim, physically fit, trance-formed body.

"Feel the power of the orange energy build your confidence and self-control to select the right foods in the right amounts that will serve you well in your quest to get and keep the body you want and deserve.

"Breathe ... going down, down, deeper down.

"Become aware now of any personal meaning the color orange has for you. How can that help you achieve your weight, size, and shape goals?"

Bob paused for a minute and then continued.

"Breathe … Good …

"Next to the orange light is a bright yellow band of light.

"Move into the clear yellow light energy and go deeper into trance.

"Sense the yellow energy flowing through every part of your slim, trim, physically fit, trance-formed body.

"Feel the power of yellow energy stimulate your intellect to make the right choices for you and experience feelings of joy in learning to create and live the active healthy lifestyle you want and deserve.

"Breathe …

"Become aware now of any personal meaning the color yellow has for you. How can that help you achieve your weight, size, and shape goals?"

Bob paused for a minute and then continued.

"Breathe … Good …

"Next to the yellow light is a bright green band of light.

"Move into the clear green light energy and go deeper down into trance.

"Sense the loving and healing power of the green energy as it flows through every part of your slim, trim, physically fit, trance-formed body.

"Feel empowered by the green energy to forgive yourself and others and to release negative emotions connected to the pain and hurt you felt. Keep the lessons, release the emotions.

"Breathe …

"Become aware now of any personal meaning the color green has for you. How can that help you achieve your weight, size, and shape goals?"

Access Your Internal Resources

Bob paused for a minute and then continued.

"Breathe ... Good ...

"Next to the green light is a bright blue band of light.

"Move into the clear blue light energy and go deeper down into trance.

"Sense the blue energy flowing through, soothing, and calming, every part of your slim, trim, physically fit, trance-formed body.

"Feel the blue energy clarify and reassert your responsibility to communicate what you want and to be open to receive what you need to express yourself in your true slim, trim, physically fit body.

"Breathe ...

"Become aware now of any personal meaning the color blue has for you. How can that help you achieve your weight, size, and shape goals?"

Bob paused for a minute and then continued.

"Breathe ... Good ...

"Next to the blue light is a bright indigo band of light.

"Move into the clear indigo light energy and go down deeper into trance.

"Sense the indigo energy flowing through every part of your slim, trim, physically fit, trance-formed body.

"Feel the power of the indigo energy give you deep insight about your body and what it needs to maintain its slim, trim, physically fit, size and shape.

"With this insight, you now realize that you have all the internal resources you need within you to achieve and maintain your size and shape goals. Allow this indigo energy to enhance your intuitive abilities to get what is healthy for you and your body.

"Breathe ...

"Become aware now of any personal meanings indigo energy has that can help you achieve your weight, size, and shape goals.

Bob paused for a minute and then continued.

"Breathe … Good …

"Next to the indigo light is a bright violet band of light.

"Move into the clear violet light energy and go deeper down into trance.

"Sense the peaceful and comforting violet energy flowing through every part of your slim, trim, physically fit, trance-formed body.

"Feel how this high vibrating violet energy opens your mind to receive the wisdom that everything you've desired, imagined, and believed to be true about the body you want, combined with your disciplined action must become your physical reality at the conscious level.

"Breathe …

"Become aware now of any personal meaning the color violet has for you. How can that help you achieve your weight, size, and shape goals?"

Bob paused for a minute and then continued.

"Breathe … Good …

"Prepare now to leave the violet band of color and move to the center of the room where the white light shines on the crystal prism.

"Notice that when you stand next to the crystal prism, you, too, are bathed in this brilliant white light.

"Imagine now that brilliant-white light flowing down through the top of your head cleansing and clearing any blocked energy.

"Your body knows what to do starting with rejuvenating every hair follicle on your scalp to restoring youthful elasticity to your entire body's skin to making the changes you want in your size and shape.

"Allow this brilliant-white energy to travel slowly down into every space in your body, rejuvenating and restoring it to its healthy slim, trim, physically fit state.

"Take some time now to enjoy these positive feelings and to sense the wonderful effects the light is having as it slowly moves down from head to toe, cleansing, and clearing, rejuvenating and restoring, creating harmony and balance mentally, emotionally, and physically.

Bob paused.

"Good ... breathe and prepare to leave your crystal room.

"Move to the door and go back into your room. Close the door and go to the mirrors.

"As you study yourself in the full-length mirrors from the front, the sides, and the back notice how you glow from the inside with the energy you received. See how clear your image is being reflected by your subconscious mind. This is now the image your subconscious mind has of you. Feel the surge of confidence that you are now equipped to help your subconscious mind make your slim trim, physically fit trance-formed body true in your physical reality.

"It's time now to go to the staircase, reach out, and hold the handrail.

"Notice how comfortably deep in trance you've become. Each time you read yourself into hypnosis you will find it easier and easier to go into a deeper level of trance so that you quickly achieve the level that is right for you to communicate effectively with your subconscious mind.

"Whenever you're in trance at any level, you will always be able to read my words to continue through the session and reawaken out of trance when it's time to do so.

"And now, ready.

"Go up to step one. Go up the stairs in your glowing slim, trim, physically fit body.

"Go up to step two. Feel grateful that your subconscious mind understands and believes that the image it now has of your weight, size, and shape is the true you and is now taking action every moment of the day and night to build and maintain this body for you.

"Go up to step three. Feeling rejuvenated, in balance, and empowered by your journey through the colors of the rainbow.

"Go up to step four. Continue to ignite your passion and courage. Feel your youthful vitality being fully restored.

"Go up to step five. Feel the sustainable surge in confidence and self-control you now have.

"Go up to step six. Notice the joy you feel every day from living the healthy lifestyle you designed.

"Go up to step seven. Feel the love and healing you get when you forgive, release negative emotions, and keep the lessons.

"Go up to step eight. Realize now that you communicate exceptionally well and can express reality in your slim, trim, physically fit body. It makes a statement about who you are inside and out.

"Go up to step nine. Now fully accessing your deep insight and enhanced intuitive abilities to do what is right for yourself to keep your slim, trim, healthy body now and forever.

"Go up to step ten. Recognize your own wisdom in making the right choices for yourself.

"Good, you're doing fine. Breathe.

"You've done well. In a moment, I will count you up and out of trance.

"If you want to intentionally go back to this level of trance in the future, you must agree to bring yourself out of trance when asked to do so.

Access Your Internal Resources

"Let's start to count up so that you can easily bring yourself up and back into the present time and place.

"One. Coming up now, take a deep breath and come up now.

"Two. Begin to move your body where you are, stretch, and come up even more now.

"Three. Wide awake and back in the present, feeling refreshed, alert, and fully awake.

"Just stay where you are for a moment while you increase your alertness. Stretch a little and adjust your posture to help become fully alert."

Ed said, "I'm still in a daze. I need to move around a bit or I think I'll slip back into trance."

Everyone agreed and decided it would be a good thing to stretch and move around a little.

As Ed, Betty, John, and Jean rejoined Bob in the living room and took their seats, they still felt a little out of it, but they decided to push forward.

Betty was the first to speak, "I went so deep into trance I felt like I was detached when I walked into the first color. Is that normal?"

"You did go deep," Bob said. "Feeling of detachment is very normal at the mid to deep levels of trance."

"How did I do that?" Betty asked.

"You've been going in and out of trance several times now," Bob said. "Every time you counted yourself down the staircase, you made going deeper into trance easier and easier. Congratulations."

"I really just knew I was floating from one color to another," Jean said. "Is that deep, too?"

"Yes," Bob said. "Having sensations of floating or lightness is again a sign of a deeper level trance."

"While we're on the topic of depth," Ed said, "I can tell you that I was perfectly content just enjoying the images that kept floating in and out."

"Oh, yeah," John said. "I was reading along and heard you ask if there were any other personal meanings and nothing happened. It was like I said to myself, 'that's nice, but I'm not doing any work. If something comes, OK, if not, OK.'"

Some smiles but everyone seemed to be too deep in reflective thought to laugh.

Breaking the reverie, Ed asked, "What color is indigo?"

"The color of blueberries," Betty said.

"And violet?" he asked.

"Like the flower," she said.

"Purple will work just as well," Bob said.

"I got the rest OK," he said.

"I've made a brief note about the personal meanings that came to me about each of the colors in my journal," Jean said. "I think I'm going to add them to my copy of the script."

"It's like you told us in the beginning," Ed said. "We're the editors of everything we're working with here. We can add, delete, and modify until we get it the way it feels right for us."

"I know we talked about it before we went into trance," Betty said, "but the feeling I got when you talked about the red energy flowing through my body was a little unnerving at first."

"That's one of the reasons I talk about it before trance so when you actually experience it, especially the first time," Bob said, "it takes a little of the edge off."

"I was fine after you said something about it igniting passion," Betty said, "It felt like it boosted my feeling of being passionate about what I'm doing. After that, I kind of looked forward to seeing how each of the different colors affected me."

Access Your Internal Resources

"Glad to hear," Bob said.

"There was something else I did that really brought out positive feelings for me," Betty said. "I imagined that there were sets of doors on the wall where each color was shining. When I moved into that color light, I opened these doors into a garden filled with flowers of that color.

"I imagined that I was in the middle of them and able to smell and touch them. It brought the energy and meanings to life for me."

"Brilliant," Ed said. "I think next time I'm going to imagine the doors open into showrooms of classic cars painted in these colors."

"I just felt the energy of the colors flowing in and out of my body," John said. "It was really fluid feeling."

"My room was round with a huge dome over it," Jean said. "The colors were so pure that they were magical to me. They were like a fine mist of sparkling energy that I could breathe and it would flow throughout my body."

"Those are all fantastic ways of working with the colors to help strengthen their individual meanings," Bob said. "What about the white light? What did you experience with it?"

"The white light part really brought strong feelings of clearing out old junk left in my body that might interfere with my goals," John said.

"That had a very powerful effect on me," Ed said. "I can't describe it, but I felt it throughout my whole body."

"It truly was a strange and wonderful feeling," Betty said. "I feel totally rejuvenated."

"As I imagined the white light coming down through the top of my head," Jean said, "I saw the colors of the rainbow light up in my body starting with purple at the top of my head and ending with red at the bottom of my body. I loved that experience. I'm sure it's because I read about the chakras and their colors in one of the books in my boutique. The sensations and feelings were just so beautiful."

"I believe what you all experienced in your journey through the rainbow of colors will definitely add an important tool for you to use to support your ability to achieve your goals," Bob said.

"Are we coming to an end of our time together?" Betty asked.

"I think so," Bob said. "I'd like to get together in the next few days to wrap up my involvement in this fantastic journey you've embarked on."

"That sounds great," Jean said. "I need some time to come out of this daze and make sure I'm clear on where we need to go from here."

"I have some edits to make," John said. "And then go through this segment again."

"I'll get things set up for us and confirm schedules," Betty said.

With that, the evening ended with work yet to be done before they get together in a few days.

Chapter 14 Win the Mental Game

The mood of the group was positive and expectant as always, but this time there was a sense of finality. Everyone knew this would be their last session with Dr. Bob, but felt happy that they were well prepared and ready to review what they learned that is helping them win the mental game of weight control.

"Let's take a quick tour of the big parts of the journey you're on," Bob said. "Who'd like to talk about the first part, which was focusing on size and shape rather than a number?"

"I'll start," John said. "As we've talked about many times, the changes we need to make are in the subconscious mind, and it works better with pictures, imagery, sensations, and emotions."

"That's why we had to create images of our size and shape," Betty said. "That's how our subconscious minds know what we want."

"And," Ed said, "the most effective way to communicate these images to our subconscious minds is while we're in trance."

"To go into trance," Jean said, "we learned that hypnotic inductions and deepening methods are the quickest and easiest way to get there."

"Even though I feel all of us have experienced the characteristics of much deeper levels," Betty said, "we only need a light level of trance to achieve our goals."

"What about stress?" Bob asked.

"Getting rid of the small things that caused me stress made a huge difference in my life," John said.

"Yeah," Jean said. "We've also changed our perspective about just how bad something might or might not be."

"Finding the silver lining made all the difference in the world to me," Betty said. "Even when I can't find it, I know it's there, and with patience, I'll find it."

"For me," John said, "I made a list of the everyday things that stressed me out at work and then just developed a plan of coping strategies for each one of the five steps in the stress response process. I can even tell that I'm much more relaxed and in control. I've written so many plans that now my favorite coping strategies go to work automatically as soon as I sense stress."

"Very good," Bob said. "Now let's talk about motivators and getting them strong enough to get you proactively doing the right things and to help carry you through the rough spots."

"I got this one," Ed said. "It's really a matter of asking ourselves why we want to get control of our weight, size, and shape. And then continue to challenge that answer with the why-type question again and again until we know the emotions and beliefs are locked together rock solid."

"Yeah," Jean said. "The emotional connection was a breakthrough for me. It really built up until I felt like I was ready to shoot fire out my eyes and at the same time I had a feeling of joyful satisfaction that I had these incredibly powerful motivators."

"My motivators got strong enough," John said, "after I challenged them over and over again. You can ask Jean. I got really defensive."

Jean smiled and nodded.

"I sometimes use two or three of my major motivators together to get enough strength to throw out the extra food on my plate," John said.

"I do that, too," Betty said. "And it's made it really much easier for me to stay on track."

"Let's talk about changes in your beliefs that at one time blocked you to beliefs that now support you?" Bob asked.

"What really made a difference for me," Betty said, "was to write the old belief really small and the new belief in large bold print. Then just like you suggested, when I read the old belief, I drew a line through it because I didn't need or want it anymore. It was a relief to get each one replaced."

"I'm glad that worked for you," Bob said. "Crossing out the obsolete belief is the type of symbolic gesture that can really impress your subconscious mind."

"I know changing these beliefs is working for me," Jean said. "I'm not as on edge as much when people come into my shop. I'm alert, but not shaken."

"She's also parking farther away from her shop and the grocery store so she can get more walking in," John said.

"You just wait," Jean said. "I've got my own powered-up motivators for doing this."

"OK moving right along," Ed said. "Remember Jean telling us how she felt a jolt when she got her subconscious mind to tell her that it believed she was imagining her true size and shape?"

Heads nodded.

"Also remember I got no response, nothing, zilch, zero?" he asked. "Now making these belief changes in trance, I got the big jolt. In fact, I got it several times."

"What did you do that was different from what you did before?" Bob asked.

"Betty and I started doing some of the trance work from memory," Ed said. "When it came time to rehearse the new belief, we're supposed to first do it watching ourselves from a distance, and then once we're successful and ready, to mentally step back into our bodies and do it again. I did the first part okay but didn't step back into my body and do it again."

"So you missed a step," Bob said.

"Sure did," Ed said. "When I put that step back in that's when I got the jolt. My whole body seemed to change from my breathing to my feeling of knowing this was the right thing to do. In fact, it happened as soon as I stepped back in and then again after I rehearsed it."

Applause and cheers went up for Ed.

"Very good," Bob said. "Rehearsing first by observing yourself from outside your body and then mentally stepping into yourself to do it again is exactly what you should do."

"Using those two perspectives seems to work best for me too," Betty said.

"I know I've said this before," Jean said, "But I like seeing myself rehearsing behaviors that might be a little scary for me from a safe distance first before I step back into myself to own the new belief or behavior."

"Tell me how you've been doing at harnessing the power of your fear centers," Bob said. "How's the retraining coming along?"

John spoke first. "Let me tell you what happened during my last encounter with the vending machine. When I looked in through the glass, my fear center went into overdrive. I felt threatened. And then I realized that my new body image was what was being threatened and put at risk. Oh yeah, that was really good. I've had no interest in that machine ever since."

"That's a very successful shift," Bob said. "It makes it clear your subconscious mind is harnessing the power of the fear center to keep its belief in your true size and shape alive and working. Great survival reaction."

"Ed has always taken care of me," Betty said. "One of the motivators that I discovered was a need to take responsibility for my own body. So when I first started realizing that I was afraid of going without something I really wanted to eat, I took a deep breath, drank some water, tightened my belt, and just pushed through the fear. That's when I discovered that the fear started getting weaker and weaker every time this happened. I'm learning that I can do this and be okay."

"And now what happens when you see something you want to eat but won't?" Bob asked.

"I've done this with so many different things now that I just don't feel any fear about going without or having to give up anything," Betty said. "And what's so interesting is that I don't have to give up anything. I can eat whatever I want just so long as I eat it in the right portion. But for the most part, I don't want that type food anymore. I now have a choice and I'm choosing to keep my great body."

"Sounds like you've done a super job retraining your fear center," Bob said.

Betty smiled widely and said, "I want this responsibility for my own body's size and shape so much because it gives me such a feeling of accomplishment."

"From what I can tell," Bob said, "you're all hitting the milestones that tell me you're on the right track."

"Could you go through the milestones for us?" Ed asked.

"Good idea," Bob said.

"Note taking time for me," Jean said.

"The first milestone is to be able to close your eyes and ask your subconscious mind to show you the body it believes it is to help you create," Bob said. "The second part of that milestone is when you get the full sensory impact along with the image."

"To complete this milestone we would experience this imagery just like we do when we're in front of the mirrors?" Jean asked.

"Yes," Bob said. "The second milestone I look for is to see your relationship with food change. You start to notice what, when, and how much you're eating. You shift from fattening foods to nutritious foods. And you have less interest in food as a comforting friend and more interest in it as a tasty bit of nutrition. Your size portions have rolled back along with your weight and are now within what they should be for your goal weight."

"All of us seem to be well on our way to getting this one done," Betty said. "Even me."

"Good," Bob said. "The third milestone is a change in your relationship with physical activities and exercise. The first thing you notice is that you're paying more attention to your posture. Your body seems to have growing urges for more physical activity. For example, you'd rather walk and talk than sit and talk. You like being on the move and are especially fond of activities that get you up and about. And, you start strengthening various muscles to get the toned look you want."

"John and I bought a book on exercising our facial muscles," Jean said. "That has really rejuvenated how I think my face looks."

"It does," Betty said. "Ed and I have started going to outdoor festivals and shows at the civic arena where we walk and walk and walk. It's great."

"True," Ed said. "We're walking a lot more now and I did start working on my upper arms. I took two of our cloth grocery bags and put a couple books in each one. I've slowly started adding books to increase the weight. I'm ready now to get a couple dumbbells so I can do some other exercises."

"Great idea," Bob said. "The next milestone is a steady progress toward achieving your weight, size, and shape goals. The before and after photos you take of yourselves will show clear and sometimes dramatic differences. Your motivation is strong. Your blocker beliefs are fading into history, as are your fears associated with eating and a healthy lifestyle. Your inner resources are doing their jobs as well. Right now I can tell by how high your confidence and esteem have become. You're getting what you want and it shows."

Even though he was still on the heavy side of his goal, John stood, smiling broadly, and turned around for everyone to see how much different he looked from when they first started meeting with Dr. Bob. He took a bow to the soft applause without saying a word. Jean smiled proudly at him as he returned to his chair.

After things settled down, Bob said, "The fifth milestone is when the entire process becomes automatic. The slim, trim, physically fit body image you embedded in your subconscious mind is now the guiding force for your eating and exercising lifestyle preferences."

"I don't think I'm there yet," Betty said. "I can still tell when my fear center goes on high alert around the bake sales."

"No," Bob said smiling. "I don't think anyone is there yet. It will take some time and at least a few to several more times going through this entire process to get the subconscious mind to give up all its eating and exercise secrets before it can go on automatic. You can't force it so don't worry about it. Just keeping doing the trance sessions and one day it will just happen. Your subconscious mind likes taking over and doing repetitive things automatically for you. That's what it's designed to do."

"It took years for us to get to the size and shape we were in when we started this journey," John said. "I think doing these trance activities is the best investment in our future lives we can make right now."

"But more than that," Betty said. "Ed and I have become so much closer in our relationship."

"Yeah," Jean said. "John and I are too. But something I've noticed when I go through the difference trance activities by myself is how much more I'm really beginning to understand my true self. John said the same thing was happening to him."

"Oh, yes," Betty said enthusiastically. "That's happening to us too. I just find it hard to believe there was that much I didn't know about myself. But what I'm learning has really helped me be much more understanding and accepting of myself. This has been a great confidence booster for me."

"I'm glad to hear that," Bob said. "I was hoping that each of you would get the opportunity to go through the full process alone and in your own time."

"My priorities are also starting to change," Ed said. "I like spending time with Betty out doing things and that's put my work in a better perspective. While it's not less important, my entire identity is not tied up in it as it was before. I'm more relaxed at work and I think as a result, I'm doing a better job."

"Personally," Jean said. "I like myself better. There were times when I was so angry with myself because I couldn't make any progress on my weight goals and that made me hard on my employees and John too. But now, I feel I'm much more pleasant to be around. At least I see more smiling faces in the boutique and John's smiling more."

"I think each of you will have more of these types of discoveries and pleasant changes," Bob said. "It just happens when you get comfortable communicating with your subconscious, which is really just getting more comfortable with yourself."

"Yeah," Ed said. "It's also knocked the wind out of my stress levels."

"As we get closer to wrapping up our time together," Bob said. "I would like you to write on your calendars a reminder to go through each of the trance sessions at least once every three months for the next year. After that, you can check yourself once or twice a year or anytime you notice a change in your eating habits or lifestyle."

"I've made a note in my journal will write down our follow-up sessions on our calendar at home," Jean said.

"So I think all of you have achieved what you've asked me to help you do," Bob said. "You now know what your body goals look like, you're getting your stress under control, you've given your motivators the power of attitudes, you've traded in obsolete blocker beliefs for new supportive beliefs, and you're harnessing the energy of your fear centers. And finally, you're now aware of special internal resources available to you to call on during your journey to get and keep the bodies you want."

"And we know how to use this process," Ed said. "With the materials, you've given us, we can drop back into trance anytime we want to fix whatever needs fixing."

"Yes," Bob said. "It's clear from your baggy clothes getting baggier that you've learned your lessons well. I can see that you are well on your way to winning the mental game of weight control at the subconscious level. That's where it's all happening for you now and in very a good way."

"It really is a series of mental challenges where we've all had both large and small victories," Ed said. "They all count."

"It won't be long before Betty and I will be just where we want to be with our weight, size, and shape," Jean said. "And then we're planning a shopping extravaganza. Score one for the women's team."

"Hey, wait a minute," John said. "What about all those clothes you have in your closet that you couldn't wear before? That's what started this whole thing, to begin with."

"New styles," Betty said. "Ever heard about new styles?"

"Bob," John said, "all kidding aside, as you pointed out we're all continuing to drop the right amount of the right pounds and we really thank you for the work you've done for us."

"Yes," Ed said. "Let me add that I've certainly changed my tune about what I believe is possible using hypnosis. I can't deny my personal experiences. Just amazing."

Jean and Betty carried on for a few minutes about all they had learned and the results they're getting.

Bob thanked Betty and Ed for hosting the sessions and then took leave of the group to let them sort out their future plans.

"What if the four of us got together in a few months to check in to see how we've made this work for us?" Jean asked.

"That sounds like a great idea," Betty said. "Ed and I are going to start back through everything to make sure we got it all."

"Yeah, we are too," John said. "Knowing what we now know, going back through the materials would probably give us a deeper understanding and greater insight about everything we've done."

"And because of that, I'm sure we'll learn so much more," Jean said.

Ed speaking to Jean said, "I know you and Betty see each other all the time so perhaps in a few months, Betty could coordinate schedules. Maybe have a dinner party?"

"That sounds like so much fun," Betty said. "Can you even begin to imagine what we'll be eating then?"

Everyone looked at each other and broke out laughing.

The night was done and the night was young. Everyone was eager to strengthen what they'd learned and to make sure they didn't miss anything before setting it aside and letting it do its work.

APPENDIX

In this Appendix, you'll find the full BLINK induction and the full body sculpting deepening staircase countdown that was broken up during the discussions in the book.

Select what you'd like to use and tab the pages, then blink your way into trance, do the work you want to do, and count yourself back out of trance.

- Blink Induction
- Deepening Staircase: Body Sculpting
- Work with the Full-Length Mirrors
- Power-up Motivator Beliefs into Attitudes
- Replace Obsolete Beliefs with Supportive Beliefs / Attitudes
- Redirect Fears and Create Supportive Beliefs / Attitudes
- Reawakening Staircase: Body Sculpting / Count Up

Blink Induction

The 'BLINK' trance induction is easy and effective. Once you've gone through the process once or twice, this is all you'll need to be able to do it anytime you want.

Are you ready to go into hypnosis?

Agree and continue.

And if it meets with your approval, will you do what I ask you to do?

Agree and continue.

Always know that should something require your attention while you're in hypnosis, you'll be able to come up and out immediately fully alert and ready to deal with it.

Start by releasing some of the muscle tension and mental distractions by taking a deep breath and as you exhale feel the tension flow out of your body.

Again, take a deep refreshing and cleansing breath and exhale. Continue to breathe deeply and comfortably for a little while longer. Focus on your breathing.

Should you become aware of any sounds or other distractions, simply notice them, let them increase your focus and concentration on this process, and then let them fade away into the background.

When you read the word 'Breathe' on your hypnosis script, take a deep breath, exhale, and continue reading.

Take your time with this.

Whenever you read the word 'BLINK' on your hypnosis script, please blink your eyes and then continue reading.

Here we go. Want it to happen, expect it to happen, allow it to happen.

Breathe.

Five, BLINK.

Feeling good, focused, anticipating going into trance.

BLINK.
No pressure, no rush, slow down.
BLINK.
Breathe deeply and exhale. Focus on your breathing.
Four, BLINK.
Slowing down.
BLINK.
Open to the experience.
BLINK.
Going down, deeper down.
Three, BLINK.
BLINK.
Focus on your breathing while you read.
BLINK.
Breathe deeply and exhale. In, out, in, out.
Going slower now.
Two, BLINK.
Wonderful feeling going deeper and deeper into trance.
BLINK.
Narrow your focus to what you're reading.
BLINK.
Breathe deeply and exhale.
Slower and deeper down.
One, BLINK.
Drifting down, feeling good.
BLINK.
Focus on the words you're reading, and let the background fade away.
BLINK.
Going deeper, deeper down.
You can blink normally and automatically now.
Breathe deeply and exhale.

Trance Formed Body

Whenever you're in trance at any level, you will always be able to read my words to continue through the session and reawaken out of trance when it's time to do so.

Deepening Staircase: Body Sculpting

Now that you're comfortable, let's start making sure the image of what you want your body to look like is clear and imprinted on your subconscious mind.

Imagine that you're at the top of a 10-step staircase.

At the bottom of your staircase is a room where you can communicate directly with your subconscious mind.

Imagine now that you're looking down at the staircase. Are the steps made of marble, wood, or are they carpeted? Is the staircase wide and grand or more narrow and bright?

What about the handrail? Where is it placed? What is it made of? What shape does it take?

It's your staircase and handrail, so you can make them as you wish.

Each time you go down a step you'll notice your concentration increase and your focus narrow as you drift deeper and deeper into trance. You can either step down or gently float down the stairs.

If you're ready now, let's start down the staircase one step at a time.

Ten. Hold the handrail and notice its texture and temperature. Take a deep breath, and as you exhale, go down a step.

Nine. Focus on your face. Imagine how you want it to look that's different than it is now. Look closely at your forehead, eyes, cheeks, and chin.

Notice the change when you remove excess fat and tighten the skin. Mentally exercise the muscles in your face. Notice how they give your face a lift.

Take a deep breath, and as you exhale, go down a step.

Eight. Imagine and narrow your focus to your jaw and neck. How would you want them to change as you remove the excess fat and tighten the skin?

Imagine them slim and trim.

Mentally exercise and tone the muscles in your neck and jaw to create the physical appearance that is natural and attractive for your bone structure. See the change now.

Take a deep breath, and as you exhale, go down a step.

Seven. Imagine and focus on your shoulders and back.

Imagine removing any excess fat and changing them to your desired slim and trim size and shape.

Mentally exercise the muscles in your shoulders and back. Feel the muscle tone under your skin. Imagine what that looks like. See the change now.

Take a deep breath, and as you exhale, go down a step.

Six. Imagine and focus on your arms, elbows, forearms, hands, and fingers.

Imagine removing the excess fat and loose skin, allowing them to change to your desired slim and trim size and shape.

Mentally exercise and tone the muscles in your arms and hands to create the physical appearance that is natural and attractive for you. See the change now.

Take a deep breath, and as you exhale, go down a step.

Five. Imagine and focus on your chest.

Notice how it gently moves each time you breathe.

Breathe.

And as your chest moves, imagine it changing to your desired size and shape.

Mentally exercise and tone the muscles in your chest to create the physical appearance that is natural and attractive for you. See it change now.

Take a deep breath, and as you exhale, go down a step.

Four. Focus now on your stomach area, waist, and lower back.

Imagine removing the excess fat around your stomach area, waist, and lower back and seeing the change to your desired slim and trim size and shape.

See your waist exactly as you want it. View it from the front, from the side, from the back.

Mentally exercise and tone the muscles in your stomach area, waist, and lower back to create the physical appearance that is natural and attractive for you. See the change now.

Take a deep breath, and as you exhale, go down a step.

Three. Imagine and focus on your hips.

Imagine removing the excess fat and seeing them change to your desired slim and trim size and shape.

Mentally exercise and tone the muscles around your hips to create the physical appearance that is natural and attractive for you. See the change now.

Take a deep breath, and as you exhale, go down a step.

Two. Imagine and focus on your legs.

Imagine removing all the excess fat and seeing them change to your desired slim and trim size and shape.

See them from the front, from the side, from the back.

Mentally exercise and tone the muscles in your legs. See and feel the muscle tone under your skin. Imagine creating the physical appearance that is natural and attractive for you. See the change now.

Take a deep breath, and as you exhale, go down a step.

One. Imagine and focus on your ankles, feet, and toes.

Imagine removing any excess fat and then seeing them change to your desired slim and trim size and shape.

Look down at your ankles and feet. Imagine them as you want them to look and feel. In your mind, stretch and move your toes. Feel good.

Trance Formed Body

Mentally exercise and tone the muscles in your ankles, feet, and toes to create the physical appearance that is natural and attractive for you. See the change now.

Holding on to the handrail, take a deep breath, exhale, and go down into the room at the bottom of the staircase.

Work with the Full-Length Mirrors

In this very special room, you are communicating your thoughts, feelings, and images directly to your subconscious mind and it is sensing, watching, and learning.

Look around the room, and notice at one end there is a set of full-length mirrors positioned at angles so that when you try on clothes you can see yourself from the front, sides, and back.

These are very special mirrors in that they can only reflect what the subconscious mind believes to be real. When the mirrors reflect what you imagine, then the subconscious mind is letting you know that it understands and believes the imagined you is real. This is the body your subconscious mind will now guide you to make in your physical reality.

Select from your open closet the clothes you want to wear in the size you want. Instantly put them on with just a thought. Notice how easily they go on and how good they fit your slim, trim, physically fit body.

With your new clothes on, imagine with all your senses what it feels like to look good in them. Feel those clothes on your body. Smell how fresh they are. Hear the movement of the material.

Feel yourself moving in them. Sense how comfortable they feel all over your body.

Now imagine standing in front of the mirrors in your room so you can view your physical image from the front, from the side, and from the back wearing your favorite clothes.

Realize that the muscle tone you've achieved helps make these clothes look so good.

Notice the improvements in your posture and how much better that makes the clothes look on you.

You believe this slim and trim person is the true you. Hold that image in your mind with all your senses actively involved.

Say to yourself, "I believe this slim and trim person is the true me. I believe this is my real body."

Make sure your subconscious mind is clear on what you want and that this is your true body. Is what you imagine being reflected in the mirrors? What you see is what your subconscious mind understands and believes you want.

Take a moment now and ask your subconscious mind to let you know when it believes that this is your true physical size and shape that it is to guide you to make in your physical reality.

Wait for a shift or feeling of some sort, acknowledging the subconscious mind is adopting your image as its own. It could happen now or a little later.

Ask your subconscious mind to guide you during your daily life on what you must do to help create the body it now believes is the true you.

You're doing fine. Breathe

Become aware and be open to the guidance your subconscious mind provides.

You are slim, trim, and physically fit, so act and eat like the slim, trim, physically fit person you believe yourself to be.

Hear yourself say, "I am slim, trim, and physically fit with good muscle tone at a size and shape that is right and attractive for my body's height and frame. I think, act and eat like the slim, trim, physically fit person I am."

You're doing fine. Take a deep breath and let it out.

Say silently to yourself, "I believe this is my true size and shape. It is me. I own it. I'm grateful that my subconscious mind can learn and do everything in its power to quickly, automatically, and safely make this the real physical me."

Good, you're doing fine. Breathe.

Power-up Motivator Beliefs into Attitudes

Write the motivators you want to use and then challenge them to make sure the subconscious clearly understands and agrees they are strong enough.

Motivator: _____
Why? _____

Check to see if the motivator is now strong enough. If not, challenge it again and again until you feel the power. Test it. In your mind, put it into action and see it work for you. Watch yourself do it from a distance and then when you get a successful outcome and you're ready, mentally step back into your body and do it again.

Imagine and experience this with all your physical senses. See it, hear it, touch it, taste it, smell it, and now own it.

Notice when it locks in.

Replace Obsolete Beliefs with Supportive Beliefs / Attitudes

I used to believe _____
But that was wrong for me.
I now believe _____
Why? _____

Check to see if the new belief is now strong enough. If not, challenge it again and again until you feel the power. Test it. In your mind, put it into action and see it work for you. Watch yourself do it from a distance and then when you get a successful outcome and you're ready, mentally step back into your body and do it again.

Imagine and experience this with all your physical senses. See it, hear it, touch it, taste it, smell it, and now own it.

Notice when it locks in.

Redirect Fears and Create Supportive Beliefs / Attitudes

I used to overeat because of my fear of _____
But now I'm more afraid of losing my slim, trim body I'm working so hard to get and keep.
I now believe _____
Why? _____

"Check to see if the new belief is now strong enough. If not, challenge it again and again until you feel the power. Test it. In your mind, put it into action and see it work for you. Watch yourself do it from a distance and then when you get a successful outcome and you're ready, mentally step back into your body and do it again.

Imagine and experience this with all your physical senses. See it, hear it, touch it, taste it, smell it, and now own it.

Notice when it locks in.

Reawakening Staircase: Body Sculpting / Count up

It's time now to go to the staircase, reach out, and hold the handrail.

Notice how comfortably deep in trance you've become. Each time you read yourself into hypnosis, you will find it easier and easier to go into a deeper level of trance so that you quickly achieve the level that is right for you to communicate effectively with your subconscious mind.

Whenever you're in trance at any level, you will always be able to read my words to continue through the session and reawaken out of trance when it's time to do so.

And now, ready.

Go up to step one in your slim, trim, physically fit body. It's yours now and forever.

Go up to step two. Feel grateful that your subconscious mind understands and believes in what you want and is now taking action to bring it to physical reality.

Go up to step three. Notice how your feet, legs, and hips look and move as you go up the stairs.

Go up to step four. Observe your stomach, waist, lower back. Watch your muscles moving.

Go up to step five. See your chest moving as you breathe. It's just as you want it to be.

Go up to step six. Notice your hand on the handrail. Watch your arms move.

Go up to step seven. See your shoulders and back, muscles toned and moving smoothly.

Go up to step eight. Observe your jaw and neck. See how they look. They are just as you want them to be.

Go up to step nine. Notice the smile on your slim, trim face.

Go up to step ten. Now mentally step back into your body and feel wonderful about the experiences you're having.

Good, you're doing fine. Breathe.

In a moment, you will count yourself up and completely out of trance.

If you want to intentionally go back to this level of trance in the future, you must agree to bring yourself out of trance when asked to do so.

Start to count up so that you can easily bring yourself up and back into the present time and place.

One. Coming up now, take a deep breath and come up now.

Two. Begin to move your body where you are, stretch, and come up even more now.

Three. Wide awake and back in the present, feeling refreshed, alert, and fully awake.

Stay where you are for a moment while you increase your alertness. Stretch a little and adjust your posture to help become fully alert.

www.ingramcontent.com/pod-product-compliance
Lightning Source LLC
Chambersburg PA
CBHW052016290426
44112CB00014B/2267